The Massachusetts General Hospital/ McLean Hospital

Residency Handbook *of* Psychiatry

The Massachusetts General Hospital/ McLean Hospital

Residency Handbook *of* Psychiatry

Editors

James Niels Rosenquist, MD, PhD
Senior House Officer, MGH/McLean Adult Psychiatry Residency Training Program
Clinical Fellow, Harvard Medical School

Sherry Nykiel, MD
Senior House Officer, MGH/McLean Adult Psychiatry Residency Training Program
Chief Resident, Outpatient Services
McLean Hospital
Clinical Fellow, Harvard Medical School

Trina Chang, MD
Assistant in Psychiatry, Massachusetts General Hospital
Instructor, Harvard Medical School

Kathy Sanders, MD
Director, MGH/McLean Adult Psychiatry Residency Training Program
Assistant Professor of Psychiatry, Harvard Medical School
Boston, Massachusetts

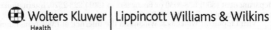

Wolters Kluwer Health | Lippincott Williams & Wilkins
Philadelphia • Baltimore • New York • London
Buenos Aires • Hong Kong • Sydney • Tokyo

Acquisitions Editor: Charles W. Mitchell
Managing Editor: Sirkka E. Howes
Product Manager: Tom Gibbons
Manufacturing Manager: Alicia Jackson
Marketing Manager: Kimberly Schonberger
Cover Designer: Steve Druding
Production Service: Aptara Corporation

530 Walnut Street
Philadelphia, PA 19106 USA
LWW.com

Printed in the United States of America

Library of Congress Cataloging-in-Publication Data

The Massachusetts General Hospital/McLean Hospital residency handbook of psychiatry / editors, James Niels Rosenquist . . . [et al.].
p. ; cm.
Includes bibliographical references and index.
ISBN 978-0-7817-9504-3
1. Psychiatry—Handbooks, manuals, etc. 2. Residents (Medicine)—Handbooks, manuals, etc. I. Rosenquist, James Niels. II. Massachusetts General Hospital. III. McLean Hospital. IV. Title: Residency handbook of psychiatry.
[DNLM: 1. Mental Disorders—diagnosis—Handbooks. 2. Mental Disorders—therapy—Handbooks. WM 34 M414 2009]
RC456.M375 2009
616.89'075—dc22

2009008850

Care has been taken to confirm the accuracy of the information presented and to describe generally accepted practices. However, the authors, editors, and publisher are not responsible for errors or omissions or for any consequences from application of the information in this book and make no warranty, expressed or implied, with respect to the currency, completeness, or accuracy of the contents of the publication. Application of the information in a particular situation remains the professional responsibility of the practitioner.

The authors, editors, and publisher have exerted every effort to ensure that drug selection and dosage set forth in this text are in accordance with current recommendations and practice at the time of publication. However, in view of ongoing research, changes in government regulations, and the constant flow of information relating to drug therapy and drug reactions, the reader is urged to check the package insert for each drug for any change in indications and dosage and for added warnings and precautions. This is particularly important when the recommended agent is a new or infrequently employed drug.

Some drugs and medical devices presented in the publication have Food and Drug Administration (FDA) clearance for limited use in restricted research settings. It is the responsibility of the health care provider to ascertain the FDA status of each drug or device planned for use in their clinical practice.

To purchase additional copies of this book, call our customer service department at (800) 638-3030 or fax orders to (301) 223-2320. International customers should call (301) 223-2300.

Visit Lippincott Williams & Wilkins on the Internet: at LWW.com. Lippincott Williams & Wilkins customer service representatives are available from 8:30 am to 6 pm, EST.

To our faculty, for teaching us the how
and
our patients, for reminding us of the why
and
our families, especially Anna, Jason and Nikki,
for their unwavering support

CONTENTS

INTRODUCTION

The tripartite mission of Massachusetts General Hospital (MGH) and McLean Psychiatry is clinical care, training, and scholarship. With this volume, our residents, past and current, have "hit the trifecta" by teaming up to create a guide to patient care; to offer a scholarly, evidence-informed resource; and to help their fellow trainees everywhere. We are very proud of these people for what they have accomplished, from before they joined the MGH/McLean Residency to how they go about their work now and for their producing this stellar text. That they came together around this project is not surprising; the defining characteristic of our residency classes has been their dedication to others through community service, care of patients, and support of each other. With this volume, they have broadened that support of their fellow residents from within our program to include all of their fellow residents from coast to coast and around the world. With this volume, not only will psychiatry residents have a practical guide and a reference for their training journey, but they will also have some of the most inspiring young psychiatrists in their pocket to accompany them. With pride, we are inspired by them to introduce this book to you.

Jerrold Rosenbaum, MD
Chief of Psychiatry, Massachusetts General Hospital
Stanley Cobb Professor of Psychiatry, Harvard Medical School
President and Executive Director, MGH Mood and Anxiety Disorders Institute (MADI)

Scott Rauch, MD
President and Psychiatrist in Chief, McLean Hospital
Chair of Partners Psychiatry and Mental Health
Professor of Psychiatry, Harvard Medical School

FOREWORD

Every July, our program's attention turns to welcoming new PGY 1 and 2 residents with much teaching, supervision, and support from our senior residents. To that end, we have a residency handbook that covers many clinical and practical aspects for a beginning resident in our program. Using this handbook as a PGY-2 resident in 2007, James Niels Rosenquist and Sherry Nykiel (Class of 2009) decided to expand the content of our handbook into a useful book that would be helpful to residents beyond our program. That began a 2-year odyssey that quickly caught the hearts and minds of the residents and faculty at MGH and McLean.

Every year, 16 residents join our program, and 16 residents graduate. Our residents come from all over the United States and other countries. They represent a unique group of psychiatry residents in their brilliance, generosity, collegial spirit, curiosity, and desire to have fun while pursuing rigorous training. This training provides them a shot at a star-studded career in academic psychiatry and as outstanding clinicians wherever they find themselves practicing. Nearly two thirds of each class stay in Boston, and we are continually enriched by their passion for psychiatry and contributions to our field. This handbook is one contribution that we present to you with the hope that our enthusiasm and commitment to learning touches you as you consult it around the clock, whether alone or with others. The heartfelt efforts of our residents imbue this handbook, and I encourage you to appropriate their wit, wisdom, and grit as you go about the task of using your clinical experiences to become the best psychiatrist possible!

Kathy Sanders, MD
Director, MGH/McLean Adult Psychiatry
Residency Training Program
Assistant Professor of Psychiatry, Harvard Medical School

EDITORS' PREFACE

It is fair to say that psychiatry is the most ambiguous of the medical professions, both in terms of diagnosis and treatment. Although this provides a particular (and to many in our field, exciting) clinical challenge, it does not mean that a careful and systematic approach to the practice of psychiatry is unnecessary. This book seeks to provide those in clinical training with a concise and accurate source of diagnostic and treatment information for quick reference. In the design and production of this book, we, as both editors and residents, have been guided by a simple proposition—what do we need most and most often? At times, our answers to these questions deviated from existing references, particularly in terms of the organization and presentation of the material. We welcome feedback on these and all other aspects of the book as we seek to improve it for future editions.

This book is the result of a large collaboration between the residents of the MGH/McLean residency program and the faculty of both institutions. Although this book has been written by residents for residents, our work would have proven impossible without the significant assistance of the numerous faculty members who served as guides to us in this project. We as residents have been blessed with these faculty who have served, with little tangible reward, as our teachers, mentors, and friends as we worked our way through the challenges of psychiatric training.

James Niels Rosenquist, MD, PhD

Sherry Nykiel, MD

Trina Chang, MD

Boston, Massachusetts
September 2008

LIST OF FACULTY ADVISORS

Our sincerest thanks to the MGH-McLean faculty, without whom this book would not exist. In particular, we extend our thanks to:

Robert Abernethy, MD
Jonathan Alpert, MD
Ross Baldessarini, MD
Rebecca Brendel, MD, JD
Trina Chang, MD
Lois Choi-Kain, MD
James Chu, MD
Hilary Connery, MD, PhD
Margaret Cramer, PhD
John Denninger, MD, PhD
Lucy Epstein, MD
Eden Evins, MD, MPH
William Falk, MD
Mauricio Fava, MD
Christine Finn, MD
Brent Forester, MD
Oliver Freudenreich, MD
Greg Fricchione, MD
Jeffery Huffman, MD
Elizabeth Liebson, MD
Guy Maytal, MD
Evan Murray, MD
Andrew Nierenberg, MD
Dost Ongur, MD, PhD
Michael Ostacher, MD
Larry Park, MD
Roy Perlis, MD
Laura Petrillo, MD
Mark Pollack, MD
Laura Prager, MD
Bruce Price, MD
Scott Rauch, MD
Joshua Roffman, MD, PhD
Jerrold Rosenbaum, MD
Fabian Saleh, MD
Kathy Sanders, MD
Gary Sachs, MD
Steve Seiner, MD
Renee Sorrentino, MD
Felicia Smith, MD
Jordan Smoller, MD
Theodore Stern, MD

HOW TO USE THIS BOOK

As in all of medicine, a systematic approach is invaluable both in the diagnosis and treatment of impaired mental functioning. This book is designed to provide an easily accessible and basic guide to assist clinicians-in-training in their work-up and care of psychiatric patients both in the inpatient and outpatient setting.

In this vein, the book is divided into six sections, roughly corresponding to different clinical settings and activities:

Chapter 1: The Psychiatric Evaluation

- Provides an overview of a psychiatric diagnostic interview
- Includes information on instruments such as the Mental Status Exam and the Mini-Mental Status Exam as well as important laboratory tests to consider in psychiatric patients

Chapter 2: Psychiatric Emergencies

- Provides information on the workup and treatment of individuals with acute alterations in mental status
- Designed for use in emergency department settings and for acute inpatient consultations

Chapter 3: Psychiatric Symptoms and Management

- Provides an overview of the major psychiatric symptoms encountered both in inpatient and outpatient settings
- Considers both diagnosis and treatment of specific symptoms

Chapter 4: Special Populations

- Provides an overview of population-specific considerations in the diagnosis and treatment of psychiatric symptoms

Chapter 5: Treatment Modalities

- Provides a brief overview of pharmacological, somatic, and psychotherapeutic methods of treatment

Chapter 6: Clinical References

- Provides brief reference sections in medicine and neurology that have specific relevance to psychiatrists-in-training
- Includes specific advice on the evaluation of research papers

Numerous cross-references appear throughout the text to allow for quick access to key material. Although the book is designed as a reference guide, it may also be useful to students and others seeking to gain an introduction to this fascinating field.

Chapter 1

THE PSYCHIATRIC EVALUATION

A psychiatric evaluation follows the same approach as any medical evaluation, with additional components designed to test for evidence of underlying psychiatric disorders. The format of a psychiatric evaluation contains the information listed in Table 1-1.

TABLE 1-1 Approach to the Evaluation of Psychiatric Patients

History

Sources of Information
Chief complaint
Identifying information
- Age, gender, ethnicity, relevant psychiatric history, means of presenting, symptoms, context of symptoms
- *Example: This is a 46-year-old married white woman with a past psychiatric history of depression who presents to the ED in an ambulance with worsening depression and suicidal ideation in the context of recent economic and relationship stressors.*

History of Present Illness
- Nature of symptoms (in the patient's own words when possible)
- Onset, duration, qualities, what makes it better or worse
- Recent stressors that may be contributing to symptoms
- Detailed questions regarding feelings of safety

Psychiatric Review of Systems
- Depression and suicidal ideation (see page 65 for more details)
- Anxiety (see page 52 for more details)
- Mania (see page 76 for more details)
- Psychosis (see page 92 for more details)

Psychiatric History
- Previous diagnoses and age(s) diagnosed
- Previous hospitalizations (where, when, why)
- Previous treaters
- Previous medication trials
- Current treaters (with contact numbers), including therapists, psychopharmacologists, primary care physician, other specialists
- Current medications and allergies

Medical History
- All medical diagnoses and past surgeries
- Medications including dosages
- Allergies

Family History
- Type of relative (relation, maternal vs. paternal)
- Conditions
- Suicide attempts; completed suicides

Social History
- Where born and raised and by whom
- Siblings(s) information (level of functioning including education, employment and relationships)

(continued)

TABLE 1-1 Approach to the Evaluation of Psychiatric Patients (*continued*)

- Abuse (see page 72 for more details)
- Highest level of education
- Past and current employment
- Current source of income
- Current relationships (married, single, children?)
- Substance abuse history: Substances used, amount, time since last use, treatment history (see page 102 for more details)
- Legal issues

Medical Review of Systems

Focus on major organ systems as well as neurologic symptoms (see Appendix I)

Physical Examination

General medical and neurologic examination (see Appendix II)

Mental Status Examination

Psychiatric mental status (see below for details)
Mini-mental status examination in all geriatric patients and when otherwise appropriate

Laboratory Studies, Imaging Studies, and Other Diagnostic Tests

First-line tests: Toxicology screens (blood and urine), chemistries, thyroid-stimulating hormone level, complete blood count, urinalysis
Second-line tests, if indicated: Dependent on particular symptoms

Global Assessment of Functioning

91–100: Superior functioning in a wide range of activities; life's problems never seem to get out of hand; is sought out by others because of his or her many qualities. No symptoms.
81–90: Absent or minimal symptoms; good functioning in all areas; interested and involved in a wide range of activities; socially effective; generally satisfied with life; no more than everyday problems or concerns.
71–80: If symptoms are present, they are transient and expectable reactions to psychosocial stresses; no more than slight impairment in social, occupational, or school functioning.
61–70: Some mild symptoms OR some difficulty in social, occupational, or school functioning but generally functioning pretty well and has some meaningful interpersonal relationships.
51–60: Moderate symptoms OR any moderate difficulty in social, occupational, or school functioning.
41–50: Serious symptoms OR any serious impairment in social, occupational, or school functioning.
31–40: Some impairment in reality testing or communication OR major impairment in several areas, such as work or school, family relations, judgment, thinking, or mood.
21–30: Behavior is considerably influenced by delusions or hallucinations OR serious impairment in communications or judgment OR inability to function in all areas.
11–20: Some danger of hurting self or others OR occasionally fails to maintain minimal personal hygiene OR gross impairment in communication.
1–10: Persistent danger of severely hurting self or others OR persistent inability to maintain minimum personal hygiene OR serious suicidal act with clear expectation of death.
0: Not enough information available to provide global assessment of function.

(*continued*)

TABLE 1-1 Approach to the Evaluation of Psychiatric Patients (*continued*)

Assessment and Plan
Items to Include • Identifying information (from HPI) • Symptoms present • Formulation • Diagnosis (or diagnoses) with discussion of differential **Plan** • Level of acuity • Recommended behavioral interventions (if any) • Recommended pharmacologic or somatic interventions (if any)

Specific diagnostic components of the psychiatric evaluation include the mental status examination and (when appropriate) the mini-mental status examination. Mental Status Exam:

- Can be thought of as physical exam in assessing CNS function
- Should address key areas of mood, thought, and cognition
- Use precise language when describing exam

TABLE 1-2 Terms Used in the Mental Status Examination

Category	Terms
General/ appearance	No apparent distress (NAD) (Normal) Posture Normal gait or gait disturbance Well-developed, well-nourished, undernourished Obese, thin, cachectic Appears stated age or appears younger or older than stated age Good hygiene, appropriately dressed Disheveled, unkempt Malodorous
Attitude/ behavior	Cooperative, engaged, friendly, pleasant Uncooperative Hostile Guarded Evasive Masked facies Apathetic Disorganized behavior Hostile or defiant
Psychomotor	Normal Agitated or restless Retarded or slowed Tremor, mannerisms, tics, rigidity or dystonia, dyskinesias Pacing, decreased arm swing Stereotyped behavior, gesticulations, posturing Akathisia

(*continued*)

TABLE 1-2 Terms Used in the Mental Status Examination (*continued*)

Eye contact	Appropriate Downcast Staring Avoids or evasive Furtive Glances Intense or glaring
Speech	Fluent or nonfluent Incoherent or garbled Mute Tone: Normal, high, low, monotonous Rate: Normal, increased, decreased Prosody: Normal, abnormal, flattened, amplified, exaggerated, staccato Amount: Talkative, reticent Style: Pressured, hesitant, slurred, mumbling, muttering, dysarthric Stuttering Accent Paraphasic errors Aphasia
Mood (in patient's own words)	Happy, sad, OK, depressed, angry
Affect (expressed emotion)	Congruent or incongruent Appropriate or inappropriate Labile or non-labile Flat, blunted, restricted Reactive Expansive Euphoric Apathetic
Thought content (in patient's own words)	Suicidal ideation (SI): Passive, plan, means, intent, impulsive, preparation, attempt Homicidal ideation (HI): Passive, plan, means, intent, target, impulsive, preparation, attempt Delusions: Paranoid, persecutory, grandiose, erotomanic, jealous, somatic, control Preoccupations or ruminations Somatic or hypochondriacal Obsessions or compulsions Phobias Poverty

(*continued*)

TABLE 1-2 Terms Used in the Mental Status Examination (*continued*)

Thought process (observed)	Linear, coherent, goal directed Ruminative, perseverative Rambling Impoverished Looseness of association, circumstantial, or tangential Magical thinking Responsive to internal stimuli Ideas of reference Thought blocking Racing thoughts or flight of ideas Disorganized or confused Word salad Incoherent Neologism Clanging Rhyming Echolalia Thought insertion, broadcasting, or withdrawal
Sensorium (observed)	Awake and alert Sedated and drowsy Barely arousable Disoriented Fluctuating sensorium Obtunded Hallucinations: Auditory, visual, olfactory, gustatory, tactile
Cognition	Memory grossly intact: Normal or abnormal remote, recent past, immediate or recall **Folstein Mini-Mental Status Examination** • Published by Psychological Assessment Resources • More detailed test of bedside cognitive testing • Useful tool to assess for dementia • Standard part of geriatric evaluation Confabulations Concentration: Good, poor Abstraction: Good, poor Fund of information: Good, average, poor Attention span: Normal, impaired, distractible Language: Normal, impaired naming, repeats, writing Vocabulary: Normal, impaired Intelligence: High, above average, average, below average
Impulse control	Good, fair, questionable, poor, impaired
Insight	Good, fair, questionable, poor, impaired
Judgment	Good, fair, questionable, poor

Appendix I: Review of Systems and Physical Examination

A complete review of systems is necessary to ensure that no medical issue is contributing to the presentation and to understand the physical manifestations of psychiatric presentations. The following is a sample review of systems to guide the interview.

General

- Tobacco use
- Rash or skin problems
- Fevers or chills
- Bruising
- Fatigue
- Self-care deficits

Head, Ears, Eyes, Nose, and Throat

- Vision problems; use of glasses or contact lenses
- Hearing problems or use of hearing aids
- Dental problems or use of dentures
- Difficulty swallowing
- Sinus problems
- Sore throat

Gastrointestinal

- Dyspepsia
- Nausea or vomiting
- Ulcer or gastric reflux
- Diarrhea
- Constipation
- Irritable bowel
- Blood in the stool
- Hemorrhoids

Genitourinary

- Frequency
- Dysuria
- Urinary tract infection
- Genital lesions
- Sexually transmitted disease
- Yeast infection
- Discharge

Musculoskeletal

- Joint pain or arthritis
- Back pain
- Muscle pain
- Use of an assistive device
- Ambulation problems
- Falls
- Prosthetic devices

Cardiac and Respiratory

- Chest pain
- Palpitations
- Dyspnea
- Asthma or wheezing
- Cough
- Sputum
- Orthopnea

Gynecologic

- Cramps
- Irregular menses
- Premenstrual symptoms
- Form of contraception
- Pregnant
- Peri- or postmenopausal symptoms
- Date of last pelvic examination
- Date of last menstrual period
- Date of last mammogram

Endocrinologic

- Diabetes (adult onset, insulin dependent)
- Thyroid disease
- Galactorrhea

Neurologic

- Headache
- Dizziness
- Seizures
- History of head trauma
- History of loss of consciousness
- Motor dysfunction
- Sensory dysfunction

APPENDIX II

Physical Examination

An excellent resource to learn and improve physical examination skills is *Bates' Guide to Physical Exam & History Taking* by Lynn S. Bickley, MD.

Components of a Comprehensive Neurologic Examination

Given the tremendous overlap between many psychiatric and neurologic disorders, it is vital that a comprehensive neurological examination is part of the psychiatric evaluation.

The equipment needed to conduct the examination includes a reflex hammer, tuning fork, eye chart or pocket vision card, pen light or otoscope (for the cranial nerve examination), wooden-handled cotton swabs, and paper clips (for the sensory examination).

Before and during the examination, it is important to observe the patient's appearance and movements and to pay close attention to symmetry (Table 1-3).

TABLE 1-3 Components of a Comprehensive Neurologic Examination

System	Test
Mental status examination	See Table 1-2
Cranial nerves	I: Olfactory *Problems with smell* II: Optic *Funduscopic examination, visual fields test* III: Oculomotor IV: Trochlear VI: Abducens *Pupil reactivity, extraocular movements* V: Trigeminal *Facial sensation, jaw clench* VII: Facial *Smile, brow wrinkle* VIII: Acoustic *Weber and Rinne tests* IX: Glossopharyngeal and X: Vagal *Symmetrical palate or uvula* XI: Accessory nerve *Shrug* XII: Hypoglossal *Tongue protrusion*
Motor	Observation Muscle tone Muscle strength Pronator drift
Coordination and gait	Rapid alternating movements Point-to-point movements Romberg Gait
Reflexes	Deep tendon reflexes Clonus Plantar response (Babinski sign)
Sensory	General Vibration Subjective light touch Position sense Dermatomal testing Pain Temperature Light touch Discrimination

Chapter 2

PSYCHIATRIC EMERGENCIES

Delirium

DEFINITION AND DIAGNOSTIC FEATURES

- Disturbance of **consciousness** with impaired attention
- Change in **cognition** or disturbance of **perception**
  - Not better accounted for by a preexisting, established, or evolving dementia
  - Memory impairment (most commonly in recent memory)
  - Disorientation to time and place and rarely to self
  - Speech and language disturbances (dysarthria, dysnomia, dysgraphia, aphasia)
  - Perceptual disturbances, including misinterpretations, illusions, and hallucinations (most commonly visual)
- **Acute** onset (hours to days) and **fluctuating** during course of the day
- Always attributable to a **medical** or **organic cause:** look for evidence in the history, physical examination, or laboratory data to indicate that it is direct physiologic consequence of general medical condition, substance intoxication or withdrawal, use of medication, or toxin exposure

EPIDEMIOLOGY

- Prevalence at medical admission: 10%–31%
- Older postoperative patients: 15%–53%
- Patients in ICUs: 70%–87%
- Associated with serious adverse outcomes, including increased mortality at discharge and 12 months, length of stay, hospital costs, and institutionalization

COMMON ASSOCIATED FEATURES

- Increased or decreased psychomotor activity (hyperactive vs. hypoactive delirium)
- Disorganization of thought process (ranging from mild tangentiality to incoherence)
- Emotional disturbances, including fear, anxiety, depression, irritability, anger, euphoria, and apathy
- Disturbed sleep–wake cycle, at times completely reversed with exacerbation of symptoms at bedtime (also known as sundowning)
- Impaired judgment

PREDISPOSING FACTORS

- Advanced age
- Dementia (see page 58 for more information)
- Depression (see page 65 for more information)

- Brain injury
- History of alcohol abuse (see page 102 for more information)
- History of delirium
- Functional status (immobility, history of falls, low level of activity)
- Sensory impairment (visual and hearing)
- Malnutrition, dehydration
- Postoperative state, intensive care unit (ICU) stay
- Prolonged sleep deprivation

RED FLAGS: If you see one of these listed as chief complaint or reason for consult, *think about delirium.*

- Altered mental status
- Change in mental status
- Confusion
- Disorientation
- Dementia
- Memory problems
- Depression
- Agitation
- Psychosis

LIFE-THREATENING CAUSES OF DELIRIUM

"Rule out WHIMPS."

- **Withdrawal** (from alcohol or benzodiazepines)
- **Wernicke's** (triad: confusion, ataxia, ophthalmoplegia)
- **Hypoglycemia**
- **Hypoxia** (myocardial infarction [MI], congestive heart failure, anemia, carbon monoxide toxicity)
- **Hypoperfusion** of the central nervous system (CNS)
- **Hypothermia**
- **Hypertensive** encephalopathy
- **Intracerebral** hemorrhage
- **Infection**
- **Meningitis** or encephalitis
- **Metabolic** (renal failure, hepatic failure, diabetic ketoacidosis, electrolyte disturbances, acid–base disturbances, adrenal insufficiency)
- **Poisons** (heavy metals, anticholinergics, overdose, intoxication, drug–drug interactions)
- **Seizures** or status epilepticus

MANAGEMENT: GENERAL PRINCIPLES

- *Delirium is a reversible condition and should be considered a medical emergency*
- Treat the underlying medical or organic cause(s)
- Address and minimize contributing factors

BEHAVIORAL INTERVENTIONS

- Acute interventions (see Agitation page 13 for more details)
- Provide orienting environmental cues (clock, calendar, names of care providers posted where patient can see them clearly)
- Provide adequate social interaction
- Have the patient use eyeglasses and hearing aids appropriately
- Mobilize the patient as soon as possible
- Ensure adequate intake of nutrition and fluids
- Educate and support the patient and his or her caregivers

TABLE 2-1 Selected Causes of Delirium

Central nervous system disorders	Stroke Seizure (postictal, subclinical status epilepticus) Meningitis or encephalitis Head trauma (concussion) Degenerative diseases Epidural or subdural hematoma Neoplasms Hypertensive encephalopathy
Metabolic disorders	Acid–base imbalance Fluid or electrolyte imbalance Hepatic failure (hepatic encephalopathy) Renal failure (uremic encephalopathy) Hypoglycemia Diabetic ketoacidosis Endocrinopathies (thyroid, parathyroid, pituitary, pancreas, adrenal) Anemia
Cardiopulmonary disorders	CHF MI Cardiac arrhythmia Hypotension Hypoxia Respiratory failure Shock Carbon dioxide narcosis
Other or systemic illness	Infection (pneumonia, UTI, sepsis) Neoplasm Hypothermia or hyperthermia Severe trauma Deficiencies (thiamine, nicotinic acid, vitamin B_{12}, folic acid) Sleep deprivation Postoperative states
Ingestion or intoxication	Drugs of abuse Alcohol, amphetamines, barbiturates, cannabis, cocaine, hallucinogens, hypnotics, inhalants, mushrooms, opiates, PCP, sedatives Medications Antiarrhythmics, antiasthmatic agents, anticholinergics, anticonvulsants, antihistamines, antihypertensives (especially beta-blockers and clonidine), antimicrobials, antiparkinsonian agents, benzodiazepines, cimetidine, corticosteroids, disulfiram, immunosuppressive agents, insulin, lithium, MAOIs, muscle relaxants, narcotics (especially meperidine), neuroleptics, ranitidine, salicylates Toxins Carbon monoxide, heavy metals and other industrial poisons, organophosphates, volatile substances, anticholinesterase

CHF, congestive heart failure; MAOI, monoamine oxidase inhibitor; MI, myocardial infarction; PCP, phencyclidine; UTI, urinary tract infection.

Adapted from Petit JR. *Handbook of Emergency Psychiatry*. Philadelphia: Lippincott Williams & Wilkins; 2004:73–74.

TABLE 2-2 Approach to the Evaluation of Delirium

History
Goal: To determine the underlying medical or organic cause Gather complete medical and surgical history Gather full medication history, including recent changes to regimen and OTC drugs Inquire about alcohol and drug use *in patients of all ages*
General Medical and Neurologic Examination with special attention to:
General Medical Examination Vital signs, signs of trauma, liver stigmata (spider angiomas, jaundice, palmar erythema, Dupuytren's contracture, asterixis, gynecomastia, caput medusae, ascites, ankle edema, testicular atrophy), signs of drug use (track marks, "meth mouth"), nuchal rigidity, evidence of recent seizure activity (tongue or cheek lacerations, bruising), pulmonary congestion, cardiac arrhythmias **Neurologic Examination** Cranial nerves, spontaneous movements, pupil size and reactivity, deep tendon reflexes, signs of increased ICP (headache, vomiting, HTN, low HR, unilateral dilated pupil, papilledema), gait
Psychiatric Mental Status Examination with special attention to:
Appearance and behavior: Hypervigilant, frightened, poor eye contact, agitated, exhibiting psychomotor retardation **Speech:** Rambling, incoherent, rapid, fluent **Mood and affect:** Depressed, fearful, tearful, irritable, anxious, angry, apathetic, despondent, perplexed, blunted **Thought process and content:** Paranoid, loose associations, hallucinations **Cognition:** Disorientation, decreased concentration, confusion, impaired memory
Laboratory Studies, Imaging, and Other Diagnostic Tests
Initial basic tests: Electrolytes, glucose, renal function (BUN or creatinine), liver function tests, serum and urine toxicology screens, CBC, ECG, CXR, urinalysis **Additional tests (when indicated):** Head imaging, urine culture and sensitivity, vitamin B12 and folate, thyroid function tests, RPR or VDRL, heavy metal screen, ANA, ESR, ammonia level, HIV testing, EEG

ANA, antinuclear antibody; BUN, blood urea nitrogen; CBC, complete blood count; CXR, chest radiography; ECG, electrocardiography; EEG, electroencephalography; ESR, erythrocyte sedimentation rate; HIV, human immunodeficiency virus; HR, heart rate; HTN, hypertension; ICP, intracranial pressure; OTC, over the counter; RPR,= rapid plasma reagin; VDRL, Venereal Disease Research Laboratory test.

Pharmacologic Interventions

- If possible, avoid using medications until the underlying cause has been determined
- Use lower doses for elderly patients and persons with parkinsonism, traumatic brain injury (TBI), and mental retardation
- First-line medications are typical or atypical antipsychotics (see Agitation page 13 for more details)

- Begin with a single antipsychotic and titrate the dose to symptom response
- Bedtime or twice-daily (BID) dosing on an as-needed (PRN) basis is often helpful
- Avoid benzodiazepines and anticholinergics
  - They may increase confusion or paradoxically increase disinhibition
  - Watch for respiratory depression and oversedation
  - Benzodiazepines are associated with prolongation and worsening of delirium symptoms
- Consider nonbenzodiazepine anxiolytics (see Agitation page 13 for more details)

PHYSICAL RESTRAINTS

- Used when less restrictive measures have failed or when the patient exhibits severe agitation or violent behavior (see Agitation page 13 for more details)

Agitation

DEFINITION

- **Agitation:** a state of poorly organized and aimless psychomotor activity that stems from physical or emotional unease
- Signs and symptoms: motor restlessness, hyperactivity, irritability, decreased attention, increased distractibility, increased reactivity, increased mood lability, uncooperative or inappropriate behaviors, decreased sleep
- Psychological correlates: fear, anger, anxiety, pain or discomfort
- Agitation is a symptom that may occur *in a variety of psychiatric disorders*
- Compare with **aggression**: overt behavior involving an intent to inflict noxious stimulation on or to behave destructively toward another organism
  - May be impulsive or premeditated
  - Most often not primarily caused by a psychiatric etiology

EPIDEMIOLOGY

- >21% of annual psychiatric ED visits (~900,000) involve agitated pts with schizophrenia (Marco & Vaughan, 2005)
- 1.7 million psych ED visits annually involve agitated patients with all diagnoses (Allen & Currier, 2004)
- Seen in 50% of community-dwelling patients with Alzheimer's disease
- Seen in 90% of nursing home residents with dementia (Teri et al., 1989)

SELECTED CAUSES OF AGITATION

- Delirium
- Psychosis
- Mania
- Anxiety or depression
- Dementia
- Intoxication or withdrawal
- Medication side effects

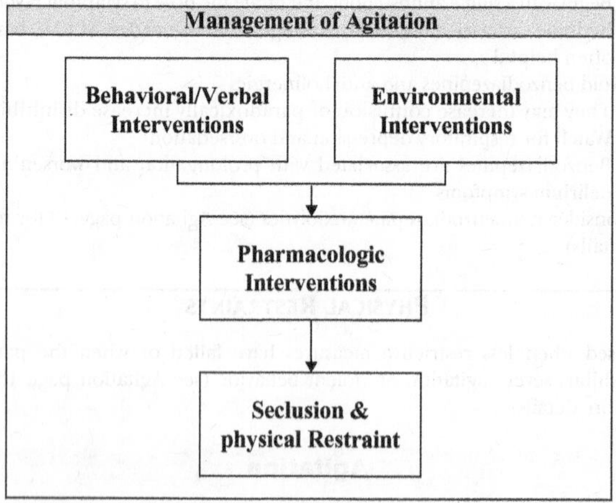

Figure 2-1 Management of agitation.

Nonpharmacologic Management

General Principles

- *Agitation is a behavioral emergency*
- Maintain patient and staff safety
- Maximize patient comfort
- Screen for and treat medical abnormalities
- Treat drug intoxication and withdrawal
- Treat psychiatric symptoms (e.g., anxiety, psychosis)
- Use tranquilizing medications if needed

Behavioral and Verbal Interventions

- Use good eye contact (avoid staring; watch facial expressions)
- Watch the person's interpersonal space (distance, altitude, movement)
- Use good posture (relaxed, open handed, equal egress, 90 degree)
- Don't touch!
- Be empathic to the patient's condition and problems
- Accept what the patient says (don't challenge)
- Anticipate shame, vulnerability, and loss of self-esteem
- Express concern and desire to protect the patient from harm
- Acknowledge the patient's power to make decisions but be firm about boundaries and limits
- Use distractions (food, drink, blanket, magazine, phone call)
- Report to patient what you observe ("you are scaring me")

Environmental Interventions

- Remove all potentially dangerous objects
- Isolate (decrease interpersonal stimulation)
- Decrease external stimuli (quiet room, individual examination room)
- Use a show of force (security)
- Provide one to one observation

Seclusion and Restraints

- These are required when patients are at substantial risk of harming themselves or others and when less restrictive measures have failed
- Always use the least restrictive means possible. Try alternative measures first. Behavioral or verbal and environmental interventions as above; as needed medications and pharmacologic management
- Implement for the least amount of time possible, as mandated by the clinical situation
- Know your specific state-mandated protocol for initial assessment and reevaluation of restrained patients
- Consider criteria for release (e.g., "able to engage in mutual dialogue with staff, noncombative"). Sleeping should be a criterion for release EXCEPT when it is thought that releasing the patient would lead to further agitation
- Morbidity associated with physical restraints: fractures, abrasions, bruises, aspiration pneumonia, deep vein thrombosis (DVT) and pulmonary embolism, decubitus ulcers (from prolonged immobilization)

PHARMACOLOGIC MANAGEMENT

General Principles

- Offer the patient as needed medications
- Try to use any sedating or antipsychotic medications the patient is currently taking
- The mainstay of treatment is use of typical and atypical antipsychotics; combine them with sedating medications or anticholinergic medications if indicated
- If the patient is unwilling to take medications by mouth or if a faster onset is required, use the intramuscular (IM) route (or the intravenous [IV] route if available)
- Titrate dose to symptom response
- Routes of administration (how long to take effect)
  - Orally (PO): takes effect in 20–30 min; maximum effect in 1 hr
  - IM: takes effect in 10–15 min; maximum effect in 30 min
  - IV: takes effect in few minutes
- Special populations: elderly patients, children, medically compromised patients
  - Start low, go slow
  - Avoid anticholinergic agents (risk of delirium)

- Give low-dose benzodiazepines only (may paradoxically increase disinhibition)
- Consider atypical antipsychotics (especially risperidone and olanzapine) in geriatric patients with dementia and agitation (*continued*)

TABLE 2-3 Typical Antipsychotics

Drug	Dose Range	PO	IM	IV	Considerations for Use in Acute Agitation
Haloperidol (Haldol)	5–10 mg	X	X	X	• High-potency D2 receptor blockade: high antipsychotic, anti-agitation effect • Minimally anticholinergic or sedating: typically used in combination with anticholinergics and BZD for sedation • **High EPS risk** when given alone (especially in young, muscular men) • IV route has fewer side effects but requires monitoring of QTc
Chlorpromazine (Thorazine)	25–200 mg	X	X		• Medium potency at dopamine receptors • Highly anticholinergic and sedating; do not need to give in combination with anticholinergics or BZD • Low EPS risk • Watch for **postural hypotension** • Do not use in geriatric patients
Perphenazine (Trilafon)	4–20 mg	X	X		• Can replace haloperidol in combination treatment • Medium potency at dopamine receptors • Medium anticholinergic side effects • Medium EPS risk

BZD, benzodiazepine; EPS, extrapyramidal side effects; IM, intramuscular; IV, intravenous; PO, orally.

Classic Combination Treatment

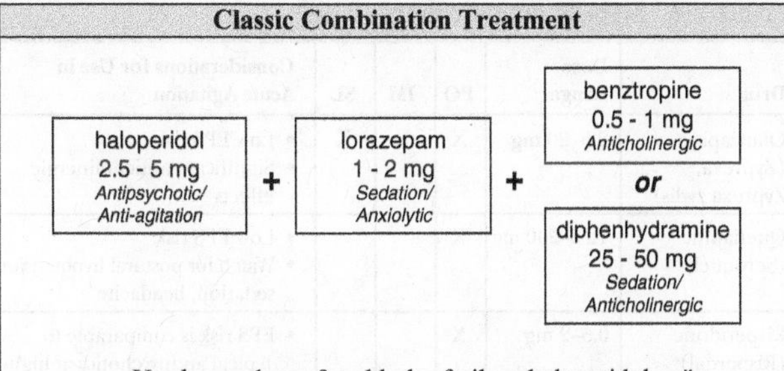

- Use lower doses for elderly, frail, or haloperidol-naïve patients or patients with low body weight
- Choose diphenhydramine for added sedative effect
- Choose benztropine for anticholinergic prophylaxis alone (e.g. patient is agitated and needs to calm down but still needs to be interviewed)
- Benztropine 1mg or diphenhydramine 25 mg provides adequate EPS prophylaxis for 12 hours
- Do not repeat them when repeating the haloperidol/lorazepam—increases risk of inducing anticholinergic delirium
- Perphenazine can replace haloperidol in the classic combo treatment when patient has allergic reaction to haloperidol

Figure 2-2 Classic combination treatment. EPS, extrapyramidal side effects.

(*continued*)

Atypical Antipsychotics

- In general, there is a lower risk of extrapyramidal side effects (EPS) than with typical antipsychotics, but EPS may still occur
- When using IM olanzapine, avoid coadministration with other medications, especially benzodiazepines or other CNS depressants as there have been eight case reports of sudden death, cardiovascular complications, and respiratory depression

Adjunctive Medications

- **Anticholinergics:** use with high-potency neuroleptics (haloperidol) to prevent EPS
  - This is especially important in young males and patients with previous dystonic reactions
  - Watch for delirium when using in elderly, mentally retarded, or TBI patients
- **Benzodiazepines:** use for anxiety symptoms, withdrawal, sedation, akathisia
  - Watch for delirium and paradoxically increased disinhibition when using in elderly, mentally retarded, or traumatic brain injury patients
- **Nonbenzodiazepine anxiolytics:** use for anxiety symptoms in patients in whom benzodiazepines are risky

TABLE 2-4 Atypical Antipsychotics

Drug	Dose Range	PO	IM	SL	Considerations for Use in Acute Agitation
Olanzapine (Zyprexa, Zyprexa zydis)	2.5–20 mg	X	X	X	• Low EPS risk • Significant anticholinergic effects
Quetiapine (Seroquel)	12.5–200 mg	X			• Low EPS risk • Watch for postural hypotension, sedation, headache
Risperidone (Risperdal)	0.5–2 mg	X			• EPS risk is comparable to typical antipsychotics at higher doses (>8 mg) • Watch for postural hypotension, headache, nausea or vomiting, rhinitis, cough
Ziprasidone (Geodon)	10–20 mg	X	X		• Low EPS risk • Watch for sedation, nausea, dizziness • Reports of anxiety and agitation (activation) resembling akathisia but may resolve spontaneously over time
Aripiprazole (Abilify, Abilify Discmelt)	2–10 mg 5.25–15 mg	X	 X	X	• Low EPS risk • Watch for postural hypotension, akathisia

BZD, benzodiazepine; EPS, extrapyramidal side effects; IM, intramuscular; LFT, liver function test; PO, orally; SL, sublingual.

SIDE EFFECTS AND MANAGEMENT

Extrapyramidal Symptoms: General Principles

- Higher frequency of EPS with typical antipsychotics
- Includes acute dystonia, akathisia, parkinsonian-like effects

Acute Dystonia

- Acute muscular rigidity and cramping
- Most likely occurs within the first week of neuroleptic initiation
- Particularly common after IM haloperidol
- Risk factors: young men, history of dystonic reaction
- Very uncomfortable and frightening for patients
- Watch for laryngeal dystonia, which includes airway compromise and is a medical emergency
- Treat with benztropine, diphenhydramine, or lorazepam
- If an antipsychotic is being continued, maintain the anticholinergic for 2 weeks (benztropine 2 mg BID for 14 days) *(continued)*

TABLE 2-5 Adjunctive Medications

<table>
<tr><th>Class</th><th>Drug Name</th><th>Dose Range</th><th>PO</th><th>SL</th><th>IM</th><th>IV</th><th colspan="2">Considerations</th></tr>
<tr><td rowspan="2">Anticholinergics</td><td>Diphenhydramine</td><td>25–50 mg</td><td>X</td><td></td><td>X</td><td>X</td><td colspan="2" rowspan="2">Use with haloperidol to prevent EPS
Watch for delirium</td></tr>
<tr><td>Benztropine</td><td>0.5–2.0 mg</td><td>X</td><td></td><td>X</td><td>X</td></tr>
<tr><td rowspan="5">Benzodiazepines</td><td>Diazepam</td><td>5–10 mg</td><td>X</td><td></td><td>X</td><td>X</td><td>RO, LD, active metabolites</td><td rowspan="5">Watch for delirium and paradoxically increased disinhibition</td></tr>
<tr><td>Lorazepam</td><td>0.5–1.0 mg</td><td>X</td><td>X</td><td>X</td><td>X</td><td>RO, SD</td></tr>
<tr><td>Clonazepam</td><td>0.5–1.0 mg</td><td>X</td><td></td><td></td><td></td><td>SO, LD</td></tr>
<tr><td>Alprazolam</td><td>0.25–0.5 mg</td><td>X</td><td></td><td></td><td></td><td>RO, SD</td></tr>
<tr><td>Midazolam</td><td>1–2 mg</td><td>X</td><td></td><td></td><td>X</td><td>RO, SD, potent respiratory depressant</td></tr>
<tr><td rowspan="6">Non-benzodiazepine anxiolytics</td><td>Clonidine</td><td>0.05–0.1 mg</td><td>X</td><td></td><td></td><td></td><td colspan="2">Often used in children
Watch for hypotension</td></tr>
<tr><td>Trazodone</td><td>25–100 mg</td><td>X</td><td></td><td></td><td></td><td colspan="2">Often used in elderly
Side effect: priapism</td></tr>
<tr><td>Gabapentin</td><td>100–300 mg</td><td>X</td><td></td><td></td><td></td><td colspan="2"></td></tr>
<tr><td>Buspirone</td><td>5–20 mg</td><td>X</td><td></td><td></td><td></td><td colspan="2"></td></tr>
<tr><td>Zolpidem</td><td>5–10 mg</td><td>X</td><td></td><td></td><td></td><td colspan="2"></td></tr>
<tr><td>Propanolol</td><td>10–20 mg</td><td>X</td><td></td><td></td><td></td><td colspan="2">Use in patients with akathisia</td></tr>
</table>

EPS, extrapyramidal side effects, IM, intramuscular; IV, intravenous; LD, long duration; PO, orally; RO, rapid onset; SO, slow onset; SD, short duration; SL, sublingual.

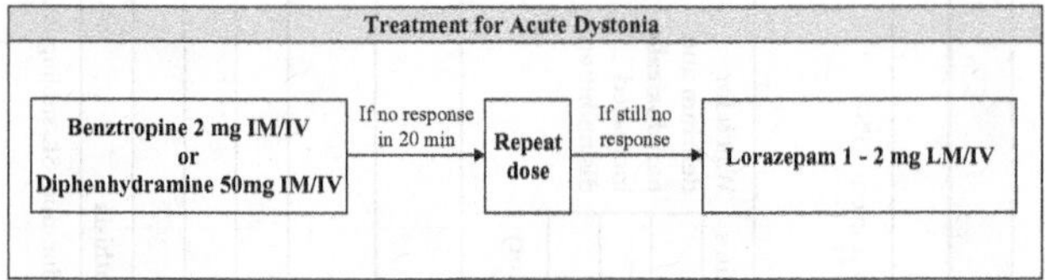

Figure 2-3 Treatment for acute dystonia. IM, intramuscular; IV, intravenous.

(*continued*)

Akathisia

- Feeling of inner restlessness and the need to move, especially the legs
- Difficult to distinguish from anxiety and agitation related to psychosis; increased restlessness after initiation of a typical antipsychotic should always raise suspicion for akathisia
- Treatment varies by clinical situation

Parkinsonian-like Effects

- Symptoms include bradykinesia, rigidity of the limbs, resting tremors, cogwheeling, masked facies, stooped posture, festinating gait, and drooling
- Onset of symptoms is usually after several weeks of therapy (*continued*)

TABLE 2-6 Treatment for Akathisia

Situation	Treatment (Ranked by Preference)
When the patient is treated with high-potency typical antipsychotic drug and does not have other EPS	1. Propanolol 10–30 mg TID 2. Benztropine 1–2 mg BID 3. Lorazepam 1 mg TID or clonazepam 0.5 mg BID
When the patient is treated with low-potency typical antipsychotic drug or an antipsychotic and a tricyclic antidepressant and does not have other EPS	1. Propanolol 10–30 mg TID 2. Lorazepam 1 mg TID or clonazepam 0.5 mg BID 3. Benztropine 1 mg BID
When the patient is treated with an antipsychotic and manifests other EPS symptoms (dystonias, parkinsonism)	1. Benztropine 1 mg BID 2. Benztropine with propanolol 10–30 mg TID 3. Benztropine with lorazepam 1 mg TID or clonazepam 0.5 mg BID
When other EPS are present and akathisia is unresponsive to an anticholinergic alone	1. Benztropine 1–2 mg BID with propanolol 10–30 mg TID 2. Benztropine 1–2 mg BID with lorazepam 1 mg TID or clonazepam 0.5 mg BID

BID, twice a day; EPS, extrapyramidal side effects; TID, three times a day.
Adapted from Rosenbaum JF, Arana GW, Hyman SE, et al. *Handbook of Psychiatric Drug Therapy*, 5th ed. Philadelphia: Lippincott Williams & Wilkins; 2005:42–43.

(*continued*)

- Most common in elderly patients who are taking high-potency drugs
- Treatment:
  - Switch from a typical to an atypical antipsychotic
  - Decrease to the lowest effective dose of antipsychotic
  - Add a fixed dose of antiparkinson drug (benztropine 1–2 mg BID)

Cardiac Arrhythmias

- All antipsychotics have quinidine-like cardiac effects, which increase the risk of cardiac arrhythmias through *prolongation of corrected QT interval (QTc)*
- Obtain a baseline electrocardiogram (ECG) or follow-up ECG in patients with:
  - Known elevated QTc
  - Family history of sudden death
  - Known heart disease
  - Known to be taking drugs that prolong QTc interval (e.g., quinolones)
- Provide cardiac monitoring at higher doses (watch for QTc prolongation and torsades de pointes)
- Replete K and Mg to a high normal range

Neuroleptic Malignant Syndrome (NMS)

(See page 39 for more details)

Anticholinergic Side Effects

- Dry mouth
- Hyperthermia
- Constipation
- Urinary retention
- Blurred vision
- Narrow-angle glaucoma
- Memory deficits
- Hallucinations
- Delirium (see page 9 for more information)

RED FLAGS: Narrow-angle glaucoma is a medical emergency leading to blindness. Symptoms include:

- Eye pain and redness
- Blurred vision, decreased visual acuity
- Extreme light sensitivity
- Nausea and vomiting
- Seeing halos around lights

Other Side Effects

- Oversedation and respiratory compromise: carefully monitor vital signs
- Orthostasis and fall risk; monitor orthostatic blood pressure (BP) and place the patient on fall precautions when appropriate

Catatonia

DIAGNOSTIC FEATURES

At least two of the following five features must be present:

- **Motoric immobility:** with rigidity, including **waxy flexibility** (e.g., resistance to arm repositioning), **catalepsy** or with minimal response to stimuli **(stupor)**
- **Excessive motor activity:** apparently **purposeless** and not influenced by stimuli (e.g., constant unrest, screaming, taking off clothes, running down hallway)

- **Extreme mutism:** verbal unresponsiveness (e.g., while occasional eye contact) or **extreme negativism:** motiveless resistance to all instructions or maintenance of a rigid posture against attempts to be moved (e.g., grinding teeth while the jaw is pulled down, squeezing the eyelids during an eye examination)
- **Peculiarities of voluntary movement:**
  - Inappropriate or bizarre posture (e.g., sitting or standing without reaction)
  - Stereotyped movement (e.g., repetitive patting or rubbing oneself)
  - Prominent mannerism (e.g., walking on tiptoe)
  - Grimace (e.g., forceful, odd smile)
- **Echolalia** or **echopraxia:** repeating the words or movements of the interviewer

Etiologies

- Neurologic or medical illness (e.g., toxic–metabolic, infections, CNS diseases, drugs, poisoning)
- Psychiatric disorder (e.g., mood disorders, schizophrenia, acute psychosis, conversion disorder)

Principles of Management

- Early recognition
- Diagnosis and treatment of neuromedical illnesses: obtain a complete blood count (CBC), complete metabolic panel, creatine kinase (often increased), Fe (decreased Fe is a risk factor for catatonia), urinalysis (UA) (consider rhabdomyolysis), urine toxicology, serum toxicology, cultures, consider brain computed tomography or magnetic resonance imaging and electroencephalography
- Close observation and frequent vital signs. Consider malignant catatonias (including NMS- see page 39 for more information) with autonomic hyperactivity and fever (associated with a 50% mortality rate if left untreated)
- Supportive care: hydration, nutrition, mobilization, anticoagulation, precautions against aspiration
- Discontinue antipsychotics or other possible culprits (e.g. metoclopramide)
- Restart recently withdrawn dopamine agonists or benzodiazepines
- Institute supportive measures: cooling blanket if hyperthermia or parenteral fluids and antihypertensives or pressors
- Suspect medical complications

Treatment

- Treat etiology (see above)
- **Lorazepam** IV, PO, or IM deltoid (first-line agent regardless of cause; 80% effective) 1–2 mg IV initial dose; may repeat q30 min, monitor respiratory rate, up to 20 mg/d (occasionally); switch to PO or nasogastric (NG) 6–20 mg total daily dose for maintenance
- Other agents: amantadine 100 mg PO BID; bromocriptine 2.5–5.0 mg PO BID; memantine 5–10 mg PO BID; topiramate 100 mg PO BID
- **Electroconvulsive therapy (ECT)** should be expeditiously used if catatonia is not responding to medications or if malignant catatonia is present

Intoxication, Overdose, and Withdrawal

Poison Control: 800-222-1222

Alcohol

Intoxication

- Signs include:
  - Slurred speech
  - Incoordination
  - Ataxia
  - Nystagmus
  - Impaired memory
  - Inattention
  - Stupor
  - Coma

Overdose

- Treat agitation with restraint and haloperidol PRN
- Treat with emesis and gastric lavage
- Provide respiratory and circulatory support
- Give vitamins:
  - Thiamine: 100 mg IV, IM, or PO once and then 100 mg PO daily thereafter
  - Folate: 1 mg PO daily
  - Multivitamin: 1 tablet PO daily
- Provide IV glucose to prevent hypoglycemia and IV fluids (**give thiamine before glucose**; see Wernicke's encephalopathy below)
- Consider hemodialysis in severe cases (blood levels >300–350 mg/dL)

Withdrawal

- Onset: 24–72 hours
- Can be life threatening
- Signs of active alcohol withdrawal:
  - Hallucinations
  - Agitation
  - Diaphoresis
  - Tremor
  - Nausea
  - Vomiting
  - Anxiety
  - Unstable vital signs
  - Altered mental status

Initial Alcohol Detoxification Assessment

- Vital signs: temperature, BP, heart rate (HR)
- Withdrawal symptoms: diaphoresis, agitation, tremor, seizure
- More aggressive treatment should be used if complicating factors are present, including elevated blood alcohol, history of seizure, delirium tremens (DTs), multiple detoxifications, comorbid history of MI, hypertension (HTN), cerebrovascular accident (CVA), abdominal aortic aneurysm (AAA), acute intracranial or gastrointestinal (GI) bleed, or spine at risk of fracture or cord compression
- Provide first-line treatment with vitamins (thiamine, folate, and MVI) as above

TABLE 2-7 Alcohol Detoxification Protocol

Prophylactic management	• When withdrawal is suspected by history • Stable VS • No withdrawal symptoms	Check VS q4h	Lorazepam: 1 mg PO q4h PRN withdrawal (hold for somnolence, ataxia, dysarthria)
Mild withdrawal	• Stable or moderate VS (temperature normal and two or more of the following): SBP ≥ 140 mm Hg and ≤160 mm Hg DBP ≥ 90 mm Hg and ≤110 mm Hg Pulse ≥ 80 bpm and ≤120 bpm • Withdrawal symptoms are present	Check VS q2h	Lorazepam: 3 mg PO q4h PRN withdrawal (hold for somnolence, RR ≤12 breaths/min, SBP ≤100 mm Hg)
Moderate withdrawal	• Severe VS (two or more of the following): SBP >160 mm Hg DBP >110 mm Hg Temperature >101°F • Withdrawal symptoms are present	Check VS q2h	Lorazepam 4 mg PO q2h PRN withdrawal (hold for somnolence, RR ≤12 breaths/min, SBP ≤100 mm Hg)
Severe withdrawal	• Severe VS (two ore more of the following): SBP >160 DBP >110 Temperature >101°F • Withdrawal symptoms are present • Altered mental status	Check VS q2h	Lorazepam 4 mg IV q 15 min PRN withdrawal (hold for somnolence, RR ≤12 breaths/min, SBP ≤100 mm Hg) Haloperidol 5 mg IV q 6 hr PRN agitation (check ECG, Mg, and K)

DBP, diastolic blood pressure; ECG, electrocardiography; PO, orally; PRN, as needed; q, every; RR, respiratory rate; SBP, systolic blood pressure; VS, vital signs.
Adapted from Repper-DeLisi J, Stern TA, Mitchell M, et al: Successful implementation of an alcohol-withdrawal pathway in a general hospital. *Psychosomatics* 2008;49:292–299.

Medications Commonly Used For Detox

- Chlordiazepoxide (Librium): 25–50 mg PO q2h PRN; contraindicated in patients with hepatic disease
- Lorazepam (Ativan): 2 mg IV or PO q2h PRN (this drug has a short half-life; it is commonly used on medical units)
- Diazepam (Valium): 5–10 mg PO q2h
- Oxazepam (Serax): 15–45 mg PO q2h PRN (should be used when hepatic disease is present)

Initial Assessment for Alcoholism

- Quantify pattern of drinking (i.e., daily drinking, amount and time of last drink)
- Medical consequences from alcohol use (i.e., withdrawal symptoms, seizures or DTs)
- How many times in the past year have you had (in one sitting) . . .
  - Five or more drinks (for men)?
  - Four or more drinks (for women)?
- CAGE Questionnaire
  - Have you ever felt the need to **C**ut down on your drinking?
  - Have you ever felt **A**nnoyed when others ask about your drinking?
  - Have you ever felt **G**uilty about the amount you drink?
  - Have you ever needed to have an early morning **E**ye opener?

Wernicke's Encephalopathy

- This disorder is reversible
- It occurs secondary to thiamine deficiency
- It is characterized by the triad of:
  - Ophthalmoplegia: nystagmus and conjugate gaze palsies
  - Ataxia: wide-based gait and slow, short steps
  - Encephalopathy: disorientation, indifference, and inattentiveness
- The disorder may consist of any combination of the above and may also include hypotension, hypothermia, or stupor or coma
- If acute Wernicke-Korsakoff is suspected, give thiamine 100 mg/day IV for 5 days and then switch to a PO formulation (especially before administration of glucose-containing intravenous fluids (IVF)

Korsakoff's Amnestic Syndrome

- This disorder is irreversible
- It is a late manifestation of Wernicke's encephalopathy
- It is characterized by:
  - A deficit in anterograde and retrograde amnesia (confabulation)
  - Apathy
  - Intact sensorium, long-term memory, and other cognitive function
- All alcoholic patients should be treated with:
  - Thiamine: 100 mg IV, IM, or PO once and then 100 mg/day PO thereafter
  - Folate: 1 mg/day PO
  - MVI: one tab PO daily
  - Check vital signs and withdrawal symptoms q4h for 24h
  - With treatment, improvement will be seen in hours to days

---

BARBITURATES

Intoxication

- Signs include:
  - Nystagmus
  - Slurred speech
  - Ataxia
  - Elevated or labile mood
  - Increased energy
  - Irritability
- Urine is positive for approximately 2 weeks after use (depending on half-life)

Overdose

- Treat overdose with respiratory support and restraint as needed
- Taking barbiturates with alcohol is a life-threatening emergency because of respiratory depression

Withdrawal

- Onset: 12 hrs to 4 days
- Can be life threatening
- Signs include:
  - Anxiety
  - Tremor
  - Nightmares
  - Insomnia
  - Anorexia
  - Nausea or vomiting
  - Postural hypotension
  - Seizures
  - Delirium
  - Hyperpyrexia
- Treat withdrawal with phenobarbital taper
- Monitor vital signs

BENZODIAZEPINES

Intoxication

- Signs include:
  - Somnolence
  - Slurred speech
  - Ataxia
  - Elevated or labile mood
  - Irritability
- Urine is positive for approximately 2 weeks after use (depending on half-life)

Overdose

- Treat overdose with respiratory support and restraint as needed
- Flumazenil may be used for acute reversal, but it is associated with a possible risk of inducing a withdrawal seizure in patients with chronic use
- Alcohol increases the risk of respiratory suppression

Withdrawal

- Onset: 24 hrs to 14 days
- Can be life threatening
- Signs include:
  - Anxiety
  - Agitation
  - Tachycardia
  - Palpitations
  - Anorexia
  - Blurred vision
  - Muscle cramps
  - Muscle spasms
  - Insomnia
  - Nightmares
  - Confusion
  - Psychosis
  - Sensitivity to light
  - Sensitivity to noise
  - Paresthesias
  - Seizure
  - Hyperpyrexia

- Treat withdrawal a with taper of the same benzodiazepine as abused, especially for alprazolam
- Switch to clonazepam as outpatient and slowly taper
- Monitor vital signs

TABLE 2-8 Benzodiazepine Equivalency

	Dosage Equivalency (mg)	Elimination Half-Life (hr)
Alprazolam (Xanax)	0.5	6–20
Chlordiazepoxide (Librium)	10.0	30–100
Clonazepam (Klonopin)	0.25	18–50
Clorazepate (Tranxene)	7.5	30–100
Diazepam (Valium)	5.0	30–100
Flurazepam (Dalmane)	30.0	50–160
Halazepam (Paxipam)	20.0	30–100
Lorazepam (Ativan)	**1.0**	**10–20**
Midazolam (Versed)	N/A	2–3
Oxazepam (Serax)	15.0	8–12
Prazepam (Centrax)	10.0	30–100
Quazepam (Doral)	15.0	50–160
Temazepam (Restoril)	30.0	8–20
Triazolam (Halcion)	0.25	1.5–5.0

OPIATES

Intoxication

- Signs include:
  - Euphoria
  - Apathy
  - Drowsiness
  - Impaired attention
  - Slowed breathing
  - Respiratory failure
  - Slurred speech
  - Pinpoint pupils
- Urine is positive for 2 to 3 days after use

Overdose

- Treat with gastric lavage and charcoal
- Provide IV fluids and circulatory support
- Naloxone (Narcan): give 2 mg IV bolus to improve respiratory status

- May repeat 2–4 mg IV bolus if no response (up to 10–20 mg as needed)
- If effective, may continue as repeat boluses or as constant infusion at two thirds of the initially effective dose

Withdrawal

- Onset: 24 to 72 hours
- Uncomfortable, but not life threatening in otherwise healthy patients
- Signs include:
  - Nausea
  - Vomiting
  - Gooseflesh
  - Nasal congestion
  - Shivers
  - Feeling cold or clammy
  - Cramping or diarrhea
  - Restlessness
  - Tremors
  - Yawning
  - Muscle aches
- Detoxification management should be provided with methadone (full agonist) or buprenorphine/naloxone (partial agonist)
- Adjunctive management of symptoms:
  - Clonidine (Catapres): 0.1 mg PO three times a day (TID) PRN for autonomic dysregulation
  - Dicyclomine (Bentyl): 20 mg PO q6h PRN for abdominal cramps
  - Promethazine (Phenergan): 25–50 mg PO q6h PRN for nausea or vomiting

TABLE 2-9 Opioid Detoxification Protocols

Full Agonist—Methadone	
Day 1	20 mg initial dose for acute symptoms Repeat in 2 hours if withdrawal is still worsening Use caution when initially dosing; do not exceed 40 mg in 24 hours
Day 2 +	Taper down by 10 mg/day until total daily dose = 20 mg Then taper by 5 mg/day until off
Partial Agonist—Buprenorphine/Naloxone (Suboxone)	
Day 1	4 mg/1 mg initial dose for acute symptoms Repeat in 2–4 hours if withdrawal is still worsening Usual total dose is 8 mg/2 mg May give a third dose if necessary; do not exceed total 12 mg/3 mg
Day 2	If day 1 dosing suppresses withdrawal, hold dose constant Otherwise, increase dose 2 mg/1 mg to 4 mg/2 mg Do not exceed total 16 mg/4 mg
Day 3	Dose half of total from day 2
Day 4	Discontinue

COCAINE

Intoxication

- Signs include:
  - Euphoria
  - Hypervigilance
  - Anxiety
  - Irritability
  - Weakness
  - Paranoia
  - auditory and visual hallucinations
  - Formication ("coke bugs")
  - Pupillary dilation
  - Perspiration or chills
  - Nausea or vomiting
  - Evidence of weight loss
  - Stereotyped behaviors
  - Confusion
  - Seizures
- Urine is positive 48 to 72 hrs after use
- Serum is positive for a few hours after use

Overdose

- Treat supportively
- Monitor for complications
  - Cardiovascular: arrhythmia, MI
  - Pulmonary: respiratory depression, pulmonary edema, pneumothorax
  - Neurologic: confusion, seizure, transient focal deficits, vasospasm, stroke, hemorrhage, dystonias or dyskinesias
- Extra caution is indicated for cardiac complications when cocaine is taken with alcohol because the metabolite cocaethylene is cardiotoxic

Withdrawal

- Uncomfortable but not life threatening
- Signs include:
  - Dysphoria
  - Anhedonia
  - Depression
  - Fatigue
  - Insomnia or hypersomnia
  - Increased appetite
  - Vivid and unpleasant dreams
  - Psychomotor agitation or retardation

AMPHETAMINES

Intoxication

- Signs include:
  - Euphoria
  - Hypervigilance
  - Anxiety
  - Irritability
  - Weakness
  - Pupillary dilation
  - Stereotyped behaviors
  - Perceptual disturbances
  - Perspiration or chills
  - Nausea or vomiting
  - Evidence of weight loss
  - HTN
  - Tachycardia
  - Confusion
  - Seizures

- Urine is positive 24 hrs to 3 days after use
- With chronic use, amphetamine psychosis may develop with possible paranoia, ideas of reference (IOR), and hallucinations. A heightened startle response, hypertensive episodes, and "meth mouth" (poor dentition) may also be seen

Overdose

- Similar to cocaine
- Monitor for hypertensive emergency and arrhythmia

Withdrawal

- Not life threatening
- Treatment is symptomatic
- "Crash" phase includes:
  - Depression
  - Agitation
  - Anxiety
  - Hypersomnolence
  - Hyperphagia

Marijuana

Intoxication

- Signs include:
  - Euphoria
  - Anxiety
  - Impaired judgment
  - Social withdrawal
  - Conjunctival injection
  - Increased appetite
  - Dry mouth
  - Tachycardia
  - Sensation of slowed time
  - Impaired motor coordination
- Urine is positive for 48 hours to 7 days with intermittent use or up to 10 days with daily use; it may be positive for 1 month in cases of chronic use

Overdose

- Treat supportively

Withdrawal

- There is no known withdrawal syndrome

Phencyclidine (PCP) and Ketamine

Intoxication

- Signs include:
  - Sustained vertical and horizontal nystagmus
  - Analgesia
  - Ataxia
  - Hyperactivity
  - Dysarthria
  - Muscle rigidity
  - Hyperpyrexia
  - Rhabdomyolysis
  - Seizure
  - Depersonalization
  - Coma
  - Hyperacusis
  - Psychosis

- Unpredictable aggression is characteristic in acute PCP intoxication; it is worsened by absent pain sensation
- Ketamine intoxication is characterized by sedation, vivid visual (and occasionally auditory) hallucinations, a sense of well-being, and decreased sensation
- Urine is positive 4 hours to several days after use

Overdose

- Treat with a quiet, dim room to minimize stimulation
- Haloperidol as needed use for agitation has not been well studied
- Avoid restraints when possible because they carry the risk of fractures
- Beware of respiratory sedation with the use of benzodiazepines

Withdrawal

- Treatment is symptomatic

TRICYCLIC ANTIDEPRESSANTS (TCAs)

Intoxication

- Signs include:
  - Drowsiness nystagmus
  - Dry mouth
  - Nausea
  - Hallucinations
  - Seizures
  - Vomiting
  - Hypotension
  - Cardiac arrhythmias

Overdose

- The initial goal of treatment is gastric decontamination of the patient
  - Activated charcoal
  - Nasogastric tube for lavage
- Confirmed overdoses usually require ICU monitoring for at least 12 hours for hemodynamic instability and any EKG changes

D-LYSERGIC ACID (LSD, "ACID")

Intoxication

- "Trips" usually last 4 to 6 hours
- Signs include:
  - Somatic tension
  - Lightheadedness
  - Mydriasis
  - Twitching
  - Flushing
  - Tachycardia
  - HTN
  - Hyperreflexia
  - Nausea
  - Restlessness
  - Excitement
  - Dizziness
  - Detached feeling
  - Euphoria
  - Depression
  - Anxiety
  - Psychosis
  - Illusions
  - Visual distortions

- Patients have a clear sensorium with acute intoxication
- Musculoskeletal injuries are common because patients have absent pain sensation, impaired judgment, and motor incoordination
- There is a risk of flashbacks with as little as one exposure to LSD

Overdose

- At higher doses, patients are at increased risk for musculoskeletal injuries
- Treat with frequent reorientation, external focusing, and calm redirection
- One-on-one supervision in quiet room should be used
- Use haloperidol and benzodiazepines as needed

Withdrawal

- There is no known withdrawal syndrome

γ-Hydroxybutyrate (GHB)

Intoxication

- Signs include:
  - Intense sexual urges
  - Somnolence
  - Dizziness
  - Nausea
  - Vomiting
  - Loss of proprioception
  - Aggression
  - Agitation
  - Psychosis

Overdose

- There is a concern for respiratory depression, particularly in combination with even small amounts of alcohol, benzodiazepines, or barbiturates
- Avoid benzodiazepines in treatment
- Treat supportively with aggressive IV hydration, antiemetics, and airway protection

Withdrawal

- There is no known withdrawal syndrome

STREET NAMES FOR DRUGS OF ABUSE

TABLE 2-10 Street Names for Drugs of Abuse

Drug	Street Names
Amphetamine	Speed, black beauty, uppers
Anabolic steroids	'Roids, the juice
Benzodiazepines	Planks, totem pole, tranks, Xannies, downers, candy
Cocaine	Coke, blow, crack, rock, snow
Codeine	Loads, cody, pancake and syrup
Fentanyl	China white, China girl, Apache, TNT, fiend
γ-Hydroxybutyrate (GHB)	Liquid X, Georgia home boy, liquid Ecstasy, soap, grievous bodily harm, easy lay
Heroin	Horse, H, dope, skag, smack, brown sugar
Heroin + cocaine (IV)	Speedball
Inhalants	Whippets, laughing gas, poppers, snappers
Ketamine	Special K, Vitamin K, Super K, ketaset
D-Lysergic acid (LSD)	Acid, blotters, microdot, boomers
Marijuana	Weed, pot, reefer, chronic, endo, dope, ganga, blunt, roach, herb, Mary Jane, skunk, fry (marijuana laced with formaldehyde)
Methylenedioxymethamphetamine (MDMA)	X, Ecstasy, E, Adam, XTC, lover's speed
Mescaline	Peyote, cactus, buttons
Methamphetamine	Meth, ice, speed, crank, crystal
Methylphenidate	Skippy, the smart drug, B-ball, jif, vitamin E
Morphine	Monkey, M, Miss Emma, white stuff
Phencyclidine (PCP)	Angel dust, dust, rocket fuel, KJ (crystal joint)
Pentobarbital	Nimbies, yellows, yellow jackets
Phenobarbital	Phennies, goofballs, purple hearts
Psilocybin	'Shrooms, magic mushrooms, purple passion
Secobarbital	Red devils, reds, Mexican reds
Rohypnol	Roofies, roach, date rape drug

IV, intravenous.

Urine Toxicology

TABLE 2-11 Urine Toxicology

Drug Class or Drug	Duration of and Result	Comments
Amphetamines	1–3 days after use	False-positive test result possible: chlorpromazine, bupropion, propanolol, chloroquine, ephedrine, pseudoephedrine, phenylpropanolamine (Dexatrim), selegiline, tranylcypromine, tyramine
Barbiturates	2–20 days (depends on drug)	Short-acting agents detectable for ~24 hr; long-acting agents ≤3 weeks
Benzodiazepines	1–14 days	
Cannabinoids	2–7 days; ≤10 days with daily use	May be positive up to 1 month in cases of chronic use
Opiates and metabolites (codeine, morphine; high concentrations of meperidine, oxycodone, oxymorphone)	2–3 days after use	May yield more true-positive test results than serum toxicology Not specific for heroin or illicit opioids Drugs that are *not* detected: naloxone, propoxyphene, nalbuphine, methadone, fentanyl, propofol False-positive test results with poppy seeds
Cocaine metabolites	2–4 days after use; peaks 4 hr after exposure	May be positive for 7–22 days after use in chronic high-dose abusers
Phencyclidine	10–20 days after use	More true positive test results than serum toxicology, but positive test results may occur with dextromethorphan

Safety Assessments

SUICIDAL PATIENTS

Epidemiology

- Among the general US population:
  - Suicide *attempts*: 0.7% per year
  - Suicide *ideation*: 5.6% per year
  - *Completed* suicides: 0.0107% per year
- 85 suicides/day in the United States (one every 20 minutes)
- 30% to 45% of suicide victims give no warning about their intent
- 95% of all individuals attempting or completing suicide have a diagnosed mental disorder
  - Schizophrenia: 50% attempt; 10% commit suicide
  - Depression: 15% commit suicide (higher in delusional depression)
  - Alcohol dependence: 15% commit suicide

Risk and Protective Factors

High-Risk Factors

- Recent suicide attempt
- Access to a firearm
- Presence of suicide note

Other Important Risk Factors

- Males (more likely to complete)
- Females (more likely to attempt)
- White race
- Native American
- Irritable or angry affect
- Impulsivity
- Frequent psychiatric emergency department visits
- Spring or fall seasons
- Access to weapon
- Change in inpatient team (e.g., residents rotating off-service)
- Unwillingness to accept help
- Soon after onset of illness or within 6 months of discharge from active treatment

Medical Risk Factors

- Seizure disorder
- Multiple sclerosis
- TBI
- CVA
- Dementia
- Illnesses with loss of mobility
- Disfigurement
- Chronic intractable pain
- Chronic medical issues: cancer, cardiac disease, AIDS, Huntington's disease, Cushing disease, peptic ulcer disease, cirrhosis, benign prostatic hypertrophy, renal disease, hemodialysis

Protective Factors

- Children in the home
- Pregnancy
- Religiosity
- Sense of responsibility to family
- Positive coping skills and social supports
- Positive therapeutic relationship

TABLE 2-12 The SAD PERSONS Scale

1	Sex (male)
1	Age (<19 years or >45 years)
2	Depression
1	Previous attempt (including prior hospitalizations)
1	Ethanol or drug use (acute or chronic)
2	Rational thinking loss
1	Separated, divorced, or widowed (recent or anniversary)
2	Organized plan
1	No social support
2	Stated future intent

Total score: 0 = little risk; 10 = very high risk

TABLE 2-13 Approach to the Evaluation of a Suicidal Patient

History

History of Present Illness
Obtain collateral information
Recent stressors
Losses or separations (e.g., death, divorce, job)
Hopelessness
Future plans
Thoughts of dying or killing self
SI: frequency, nature, severity, context, recent increase?
For SI/SA, assess:

- **Action** (impulsive vs. premeditated)
- **Intent** (examine thoughts in detail; passive vs. active)
- **Plan** (preparation, feasibility, rehearsed, left note)
- **Lethality** (including patient's understanding of lethality)
- **Method** (jumping or shooting)
- **Means** (able to obtain weapon, pills, knife, access to firearms)
- **Current reaction** (relieved, ashamed of thoughts)
- **Deterring factors** (what prevented the patient from acting)

Past Psychiatric History
Past attempts: lethality, circumstances
Aborted attempts (e.g., driving to bridge, but not jumping)
Self-injurious behaviors (cutting or burning)
Substance abuse
Panic attacks or severe anxiety

Social History
Support system
Childhood trauma

Family History
Suicides (meaning and relationship to patient)

General Medical and Neurologic Examination with special attention to:

Signs and symptoms of toxic overdose or intoxication

(continued)

TABLE 2-13 Approach to the Evaluation of a Suicidal Patient (*continued*)

Psychiatric Mental Status Examination with special attention to:
Anxiety, agitation, fear (decreased fear before an attempt) Delirium or intoxication Restlessness or akathisia Severity of mood/anxiety symptoms Psychosis Impulsivity or poor judgment Cognitive style (tunnel vision, close-mindedness)
Laboratory Studies, Imaging, and other Diagnostic Tests
First line: urine toxicology

SA, suicide attempt; SI, suicidal ideation.

Interventions

- After a suicide attempt (injury or ingestion), the patient should be seen by medical team as soon as possible and monitored closely
- Ensure a safe environment (change to hospital gown; remove sharp and dangerous objects; secure the patient's belongings, including medications; provide one-on-one observation)
- Treat co-occurring symptoms first (patients who are agitated, aggressive, psychotic, or have severe mood symptoms; use medications or restraints as necessary)
- Reassess intoxicated patients when they are sober
- Obtain collateral (family, roommates, all treaters)
- Provide psychoeducation to the patient

Discharge Checklist

- Access to means of suicide removed
- Precipitants addressed
- Underlying psychiatric illness, including substance abuse, treated
- Increased outpatient supports
- Close follow-up arranged
- Document risk assessment, decision making, and communication with treaters.

There is no evidence that "contracts for safety" are effective in reducing suicide attempts.

HOMICIDAL PATIENTS

Risk Factors

- Homicide is the second leading cause of death among people ages 15 to 24 years
- The best predictor of violence is a history of violent behavior
- 50% of individuals who commit homicides or exhibit assaultive behavior consumed alcohol before the violent act

- Patients with schizophrenia are no more likely than general population to commit homicide (but when it occurs, it may be for unpredictable or bizarre reasons)

Management

- Use restraints, seclusion, and medication if necessary (see Agitation page 13 for more details)
- Hospitalize when acute
- If expressed toward a *specific* person, the Tarasoff ruling applies: Mental health professionals have the duty to protect (not just warn) identifiable, endangered third parties from imminent threats of serious harm by patients (can include involving the police and involuntary hospitalization if necessary)

TABLE 2-14 Predictors of Dangerousness Toward Others (Include in Documentation)

Demographic	Age 15–24 years Low SES Male gender
Cognitive	Low intelligence Neurologic impairment
Personality	Psychopathology Impulsivity History of loss of control Chronic anger Hostility or resentment Lack of compassion Resentful of authority History of being antisocial or withdrawn Poor self-esteem
Criminal history	Prior violence Young age at first offense
Social history	Employment or housing instability Poor social support Low education level Early loss of parent Childhood brutality Past fire setting, bedwetting, or cruelty to animals
Psychiatric history	Major mental illness Hallucinations or delusions involving homicidal violence Active psychosis Current substance abuse
Situation	Frequent and open threats Concrete plan Access to weapons Presence of victim Similar context to previous violence

SES, socioeconomic status.

- For a history of violence, assess and document:
  - Circumstances of past violence (target, motive, events)
  - Mental status at the time (including substance use)
  - Outcome of the violence (status of victim, detailed legal history)
  - Current attitude towards the incident (regret, remorse)

Life-Threatening Side Effects

Neuroleptic Malignant Syndrome

Definition

- This is an idiopathic, life-threatening complication of treatment with antipsychotic drugs or other agents that block dopamine signaling or sudden withdrawal of dopamine agents
- It is characterized by fever, severe muscle rigidity, autonomic instability, and mental status changes

EPIDEMIOLOGY

- Incidence: 0.01%–0.02% of patients treated with antipsychotics
- 2000 cases diagnosed annually

Differential Diagnosis

- CNS infections: encephalitis, meningitis, brain abscess, sepsis
- Psychiatric or neurologic: agitated delirium, benign EPS, nonconvulsive status epilepticus, structural lesions
- Toxic or pharmacologic: malignant hyperthermia, serotonin syndrome, central anticholinergic syndrome, amphetamine or hallucinogen abuse
- Endocrine: thyrotoxicosis, pheochromocytoma
- Environmental: heat stroke

RED FLAGS: Risk factors for NMS

- Organic brain abnormalities
- Low serum iron levels
- Dehydration
- Concomitant use of lithium
- Simultaneous administration of multiple neuroleptics
- Most common with typical antipsychotics, but does occur with atypicals

Treatment

- Prompt removal of causative agent (or if NMS has been caused by discontinuation of dopaminergic therapy, urgent reinstitution)
- ICU for close vital signs and hemodynamic monitoring, support, and treatment
- **Supportive measures:**
  - Intravascular resuscitation with IVF, nutrition
  - Temperature reduction with ice packs and cooling blankets
  - Respiratory support with ventilation if necessary
  - Prophylaxis of ARF secondary to rhabdomyolysis with IVF, urine alkalinization, hemodialysis if necessary
  - DVT prophylaxis with heparin or pneumoboots
- **Pharmacologic treatments:** there is no general consensus on which treatment is best; this treatment should complement supportive care; it should be individualized and based empirically on the character, duration, severity, and stage of clinical signs and symptoms
  - Dantrolene: 1–3 mg/kg/day divided four times a day (QID)
  - Bromocriptine: start dose 2.5 mg TID; increase as tolerated to 5–10 mg TID
  - Lorazepam: 1–2 mg q4–6 hrs

- ECT: effective if symptoms refractory to supportive care and pharmacotherapy or if idiopathic malignant catatonia cannot be excluded
  - Six to 10 treatments with bilateral electrode placement *(continued)*

TABLE 2-15 Approach to the Evaluation of Neuroleptic Malignant Syndrome

History
Source Patient, family, medication records, caregivers **Presenting symptoms** Altered mental status, muscle rigidity, tremor, hyperthermia, autonomic instability **Associated with *withdrawal* of the following medications:** Levodopa ± carbidopa COMT inhibitors (tolcapone, entacapone) Dopamine agonists (bromocriptine, pergolide, ropinirole, pramipexole, cabergoline, apomorphine) Amantadine **Associated with *introduction* of the following medications:** Typical antipsychotics (i phenothiazines), butyrophenones, thiothixenes Atypical antipsychotics (clozapine) Antiemetics: metoclopramide, droperidol, prochlorperazine, promethazine Rare cases with TCAs, citalopram, amphetamines, cocaine, loxapine, diatrizoate, and lithium overdoses **Course** Evolves over 24–72 hours after exposure; slower onset is possible for depot neuroleptics Lasts 7–10 days in uncomplicated cases; lasts longer for depot neuroleptics
General Medical and Neurologic Examination with special attention to:
Motor symptoms: rigidity ("lead pipe"), akinesia, bradykinesia; less commonly dystonia, mutism, dysarthria, involuntary movements **Hyperthermia:** temperature >38°C **Autonomic instability:** tachycardia, diaphoresis, labile BP, tachypnea, mydriasis, sialorrhea, incontinence
Psychiatric Mental Status Examination with special attention to:
Altered mental status: ranges from confusion or delirium to stupor or coma
Laboratory Studies, Imaging, and Other Diagnostic Tests
↑WBC count ± left shift ↑CK ± ↑aldolase, LDH, AST, ALT, alkaline phosphatase ↑Serum creatinine and BUN, proteinuria, myoglobinuria ↓Ca, ↓Fe, ↑serum Osm

ALT, alanine aminotransferase; AST, aspartate aminotransferase; BP, blood pressure; BUN, blood urea nitrogen; CK, creatinine kinase; COMT, catechol-O-methyl transferase; LDH, lactate dehydrogenase; TCA, tricyclic antidepressant; WBC, white blood cell.

(*continued*)

Complications

- Renal failure
- Thromboembolism
- Multiple system failure
- Residual catatonia
- Death

Prognosis

- The mortality rate is 10%
- Recurrence is as high as 30% of patients after antipsychotic rechallenge
  - Allow 2 weeks after recovery from NMS before rechallenge
  - Restart with low doses of low-potency typical antipsychotic or atypical antipsychotic
  - Monitor for early signs of NMS

SEROTONIN SYNDROME

Definition

- Potentially life-threatening, predictable (i.e., non-idiopathic) adverse drug reaction resulting from excess CNS and peripheral serotonergic agonism secondary to therapeutic drug use, intentional self-poisoning, or inadvertent drug–drug interaction
- Clinical triad (presentation varies):
  - Neuromuscular: hyperreflexia, inducible clonus, myoclonus, ocular clonus, spontaneous clonus, peripheral hypertonicity, shivering
  - Autonomic instability: tachycardia, mydriasis, diaphoresis, bowel sounds, diarrhea
  - Mental status changes: agitation, delirium

EPIDEMIOLOGY

- 14%–16% in patients who overdose on SSRIs
- In 2002: 93 deaths and >7300 toxic effects

Drugs Associated with Serotonin Syndrome

- Selective serotonin reuptake inhibitors (SSRIs)
- Other antidepressant drugs: serotonin and norepinephrine reuptake inhibitors (SNRIs), norepinephrine and dopamine reuptake inhibitors (NDRIs), TCAs
- Monoamine oxidase inhibitors (MAOIs)
- Mood stabilizers: valproic acid, lithium
- Analgesics: meperidine, fentanyl, tramadol, pentazocine
- Antiemetic agents: ondansetron, granisetron, metoclopramide
- Antimigraine drug: sumatriptan
- Bariatric drug: sibutramine
- Antibiotic: linezolid
- Antiviral: ritonavir
- Over-the-counter drug: dextromethorphan

- Drugs of abuse: methylenedioxymethamphetamine (MDMA), LSD, 5-methoxydiisopropyltryptamine, Syrian rue
- Dietary or herbal supplements: tryptophan, St. John's wort, ginseng

Drug Interactions Associated with Severe Serotonin Syndrome

- Any combination of the following: sertraline, fluoxetine, fluvoxamine, paroxetine, citalopram, nefazodone, buspirone, clomipramine, venlafaxine, phenelzine, isocarboxazid, valproic acid, meperidine, fentanyl, tramadol, pentazocine lactate, ondansetron, metoclopramide, sumatriptan, sibutramine, linezolid, ritonavir, tranylcypromine, imipramine, mirtazapine
- Phenelzine and meperidine
- Tranylcypromine and imipramine
- Phenelzine and SSRIs
- Paroxetine and buspirone
- Linezolid and citalopram
- Moclobemide and SSRIs
- Tramadol, venlafaxine, and mirtazapine (*continued*)

TABLE 2-16 Clinical Characteristics of Serotonin Syndrome and Similar Clinical Conditions

	Serotonin Syndrome	Anticholinergic Poisoning	Neuroleptic Malignant Syndrome	Malignant Hyperthermia
Medication history	Serotonergic drug	Anticholinergic agent	Dopamine antagonist	Inhalational anesthesia
Time until onset	<12 hr	<12 hr	1–3 days	30 min–24 hr
Vital signs	↑BP, ↑HR, ↑RR, ↑Temperature (>41.1°C)	↑BP (mild), ↑HR, ↑RR, ↑Temperature (<38.8°C)	↑BP, ↑HR, ↑RR, ↑Temperature (>41.1°C)	↑BP, ↑HR, ↑RR, ↑Temperature (≤46°C)
Pupils	Dilation	Dilation	Normal	Normal
Mucosa	Sialorrhea	Dry	Sialorrhea	Normal
Skin	Diaphoresis	Erythema; hot and dry	Pallor, diaphoresis	Mottled, diaphoresis
Bowel sounds	↑↑↑	↓ or absent	↓ or ↔	↓
NM tone	↑, especially in LE	Normal	↑↑↑, "lead-pipe" rigidity in all muscle groups	↑↑↑"Rigor mortis"–like rigidity
Reflexes	↑↑ Clonus	Normal	Bradyreflexia	Hyporeflexia
Mental Status	Agitation, coma	Agitated delirium	Stupor, alert, mutism, coma	Agitation

BP, blood pressure; HR, heart rate; LE= lower extremity; NM, neuromuscular; RR, respiratory rate. Adapted from Boyer EW, Shannon M: The serotonin syndrome. *N Engl J Med* 2005;352: 1112–1120.

TABLE 2-17 Approach to the Evaluation of Serotonin Syndrome

History
Source Patient, family, medication records, caregivers **History** Use of prescription and OTC drugs, illicit substances, dietary supplements Evolution of symptoms and rate of change **Presenting symptoms** Neuromuscular, autonomic instability, mental status changes **Course** Rapid onset, within minutes of medication change or self-poisoning (60% of patients with serotonin syndrome present within 6 hr after initial medication use, dosing change, or overdose)
General Medical and Neurologic Examination with special attention to:
Mild: tachycardia, autonomic findings (shivering, diaphoresis, mydriasis), neurologic findings (intermittent myoclonus, tremor, hyperreflexia) **Moderate:** VS abnormalities (tachycardia, hypertension, hyperthermia), elevated core temperature (≤40°C or 104°F), mydriasis, hyperactive bowel sounds, diaphoresis, hyperreflexia and clonus in LE > UE, horizontal ocular clonus, mental status changes (see below) **Severe:** hypertension and tachycardia leading to shock, muscular rigidity and hypertonicity, laboratory abnormalities (see below)
Psychiatric Mental Status Examination with special attention to:
Hypervigilance, pressured speech **Altered mental status**: agitation, delirium, coma
Laboratory Studies, Imaging, and Other Diagnostic Tests
Tests are nonspecific In severe cases, can have evidence of metabolic acidosis; disseminated intravascular coagulation; ↑CK, ALT, AST, serum creatinine, and BUN

ALT, alanine aminotransferase; AST, aspartate aminotransferase; BUN, blood urea nitrogen; CK, creatinine kinase; LE, lower extremity; OTC, over the counter; UE, upper extremity; VS, vital signs.

(continued)

Differential Diagnosis

- Anticholinergic poisoning
- Neuroleptic malignant syndrome
- Malignant hyperthermia

Treatment

- Prompt removal of causative agent
- Guided by the severity of the illness
- Mild: supportive care: IVF hydration, monitoring and correction of vital signs, removal of causative agent, treatment of agitation with benzodiazepines (avoid physical restraints because they may worsen muscle contractions)
- Moderate: correction of all cardiorespiratory and thermal abnormalities, 5-HT_{2A} antagonists

- Cyproheptadine (PO or nasogastic tube (NGT))
  - 12–32 mg/24h binds 85% to 95% of serotonin receptors
  - Initial dose of 12 mg and then 2 mg q2h if symptoms persist
  - Maintenance dosing is 8 mg q6h
- Consider atypical antipsychotics with 5-HT_{2A} antagonist activity (i.e., olanzapine)
- Severe: above therapies with the addition of immediate sedation, neuromuscular paralysis with nonpolarizing agents (e.g., vecuronium), and endotracheal intubation

Prognosis

- Most cases resolve within 24 hours of initiation of therapy and discontinuation of offending agent
- Prevention is by avoidance of multidrug regimens

Lithium Toxicity

Definition

- This is primarily a clinical diagnosis for which serum levels provide confirmation
- Lithium has low therapeutic index (target plasma levels, 0.8–1.0 mM), and toxicity can occur even at levels within the therapeutic range
- Signs and symptoms of toxicity include vomiting and diarrhea, deteriorating renal function, cardiac arrhythmias, and central and peripheral nervous system changes

Red Flags: The most common cause of toxicity in compliant patients is **alteration in sodium balance.** Anything that leads to sodium depletion will elevate lithium levels.

Predisposing Factors

- History of lithium intoxication
- Advanced age
- Overdose
- Diet or GI disturbances: anorexia, diarrhea, vomiting, decreased dietary sodium intake, dehydration
- Comorbid medical conditions: heart disease, hypertension, atherosclerosis, renal damage, renal insufficiency or renal failure, brain disorders, hypothyroid
- Drug therapies

Treatment: General Principles

Red Flags: Lithium is leached out of tissues (fat), so levels increase again after dialysis. Treatment may require several courses of dialysis (especially in chronic overdose).

- Hold the next dose until the patient's lithium level can be checked
- Send a lithium level immediately
- Toxicity correlates poorly with lithium level
  - Any level above 2.0 requires treatment even if the patient appears well
  - All patients with signs or symptoms of toxicity require treatment, regardless of level
- Treat immediately; damage is caused by high level and the duration of a high level *(continued)*

TABLE 2-18 Drug Interactions with Lithium

Interactions that INCREASE lithium level	NSAIDs Diuretics: thiazides, spironolactone, triamterene, ethacrynic acid Antibiotics: metronidazole, tetracycline ACE inhibitors Carbamazepine Clonazepam Enalapril Fluoxetine
Interactions that DECREASE lithium level	Acetazolamide Theophylline, aminophylline Caffeine (mild effect) Osmotic diuretics Sodium bicarbonate Sodium chloride Urea Mannitol

ACE, angiotensin-converting enzyme; NSAID, nonsteroidal antiinflammatory drug.
Adapted from Rosenbaum JF, Arana GW, Hyman SE, et al: *Handbook of Psychiatric Drug Therapy*, 5th ed. Philadelphia: Lippincott Williams & Wilkins; 2005:148.

TABLE 2-19 Approach to the Evaluation of Lithium Toxicity

History
Source Patient, family, medication records, caregivers **Presenting symptoms** **Gastrointestinal:** vomiting, diarrhea **Renal:** renal insufficiency, polyuria, polydipsia, acute renal failure **Cardiovascular:** syncope, dizziness, worsening cardiac function, sick sinus syndrome, bradycardia, atrial or ventricular arrhythmias, SA block, AV block, junctional rhythms, bundle branch block, ventricular tachycardia, ventricular fibrillation, myocarditis, death **Neurologic:** drowsiness, fatigue, apathy, lethargy, altered mental status, seizures
General Medical and Neurologic Examination with special attention to:
Cardiovascular: bradycardia, tachycardia, arrhythmias **Neurologic**: cerebellar symptoms (ataxia, dysarthria, unsteady gait, lack of coordination), coarse tremors, hyperreflexia, nystagmus, muscle fasciculations
Psychiatric Mental Status Examination with special attention to:
Altered mental status: confusion, delirium, coma, hallucinations
Laboratory Studies, Imaging, and Other Diagnostic Tests
Lithium level ↑BUN, ↑creatinine

AV, atrioventricular; BUN, blood urea nitrogen; SA, sinoatrial.

(continued)

- In overdose cases in which the drug was taken less than 4 hours before treatment, induction of vomiting or gastric lavage may be warranted
- Consult renal and medicine services for possible hemodialysis
- The goal of dialysis is to dialyze off all lithium (level of 0)

Prognosis

- Survivors of serious toxicity may suffer permanent cerebellar ataxia and severe permanent anterograde amnesia

TABLE 2-20 Treatment of Lithium Toxicity

Level	Clinical Picture	Treatment
<3.0	With mild symptoms: lethargy, fatigue, weakness, coarse tremor, mild nausea	1. NS at 150–200 cc/hr and IV furosemide until level normalizes. 2. Correct electrolyte abnormalities, especially K+. 3. Avoid charcoal (does not bind lithium). 4. Hold lithium and work up cause of toxicity.
3.0–4.0	With no symptoms or mild or moderate symptoms: nausea, vomiting, mild ataxia, dysarthria, incoordination, hyperreflexia, poor concentration, fasciculations	In patients with normal cardiac and renal function (able to tolerate volume load): 1. Call renal consult for possible hemodialysis and treat as above while awaiting consult. 2. Check lithium levels q 2 hr to be sure they are decreasing. 3. Consider ICU transfer.
3.0–4.0	With severe symptoms: delirium, ataxia, seizures, renal failure, hallucinations, coma	1. Dialysis required (hemodialysis best but peritoneal can be used). 2. Move patient to ICU for hemodynamic monitoring. 3. Re-equilibration occurs; retest levels several times after dialysis. 4. Work up cause of toxicity.
>4.0	With no symptoms, mild symptoms, or moderate symptoms	1. IV NS at 250 cc/hr; recheck level every hour. 2. If level does not begin to decrease in 2–3 hours, institute dialysis regardless of the patient's clinical appearance. 3. Work up cause of toxicity.
>4.0	With severe symptoms	Same as 3.0–4.0 with severe symptoms above.

ICU, intensive care unit; IV, intravenous; NS, normal saline.

Capacity Evaluation and Informed Consent

DEFINITION

- Capacity vs. competence:
  Capacity: an individual's clinical ability to make an informed decision about a specific question or set of questions
  Competence: a legal status determined by the court
- Capacity is assessed clinically- *Any licensed physician* can make a determination of capacity
- Capacity is most often called into question when a patient refuses to accept medical treatment seeks to sign out against medical advice (AMA), or needs to consent for a procedure
- There must be a specific question from the team that requires addressing capacity (e.g., Can the patient refuse IV antibiotics? Can the patient consent for appendectomy?)
- The level of capacity required is based on comparing the risks and benefits of treatment and the patient's choice
- The standard for capacity *increases* if the decision does not match the presumed risk/benefit ratio (e.g., less capacity is required to refuse to clip a hangnail than to refuse repair of a ruptured aortic aneurysm)

HOW TO DOCUMENT CAPACITY

"Based upon my evaluation of this patient, he/she does/does not express a consistent preference regarding the proposed treatment, does/does not have a factual understanding of the current situation as evidenced by [give example], does/does not appreciate the risks and benefits of treatment and nontreatment, and is able/unable to rationally manipulate information to make a decision as evidenced by [give example]. Therefore, in my opinion, this patient has/lacks the capacity to make this medical decision."

If capacity is present, note:

"We should respect the patient's right to make this decision to [insert details of what the patient has capacity to decide]."

If lacking capacity, note:

"A substitute decision maker must be found for this patient using the following framework:

1. If the patient has a health care proxy, the agent should be contacted.
2. If there is no Health Care Proxy, efforts should be made to identify an appropriate substitute decision maker (most commonly a family member or members), with the understanding that ultimately, it may be necessary to have a guardian appointed in order to facilitate legal decision making.
3. In the case of a true emergency, treatment may be provided without consent, but should be discussed with the Office of General Counsel as soon as possible.

NOTE: In the three situations above, attempts to contact a substituted decision maker or the Office of General Counsel should not delay the delivery of emergent care where such delay would compromise the patient's well-being."

TABLE 2-21 Criteria for Decision-Making Capacity and Approaches to Assessment of the Patient

Criteria	Patient Should Be Able To Do the Following:	Sample Questions
Communicate a choice	Indicate a preferred treatment. *Frequent reversal of choice attributable to psychiatric or neurologic conditions may indicate lack of capacity.*	Have you decided whether to follow your doctor's [or my] recommendation for treatment? Can you tell me what that decision is? [If no decision] What is making it hard for you to decide?
Understand the relevant information	Grasp the fundamental meaning of information communicated by physicians. *Encourage the patient to paraphrase disclosed information regarding his or her medical condition and treatment.*	Please tell me in your own words what your doctor has [or I have] told you about: The problem with your health now. The recommended treatment. The possible risks and benefits of the treatment. Any alternative treatments and their risks and benefits. The risks and benefits of no treatment.
Appreciate the situation and its consequences	Acknowledge the patient's medical condition and the likely consequences of treatment options *Ask the patient to describe his or her views of the medical condition, proposed treatment, and likely outcome.*	What do you believe is wrong with your health now? Do you believe that you need some kind of treatment? What is treatment likely to do for you? What makes you believe it will have that effect? What do you believe will happen if you are not treated? Why do you think your doctor has [or I have] recommended this treatment?
Reason about treatment options	Engage in a rational process of manipulating the relevant information. *Ask the patient to compare treatment options and consequences and to offer reasons for selection of option. Note: Patients have the right to make "unreasonable" choices.*	How did you decide to accept/to reject the recommended treatment? What makes [chosen option] better than [alternative option]?

IMPACT OF CAPACITY EVALUATION

- Patients lacking capacity may require appointment of a guardian
- If there is a lack of capacity in an emergency, take appropriate life-saving action and then seek substituted judgment for other decisions
- If there is a lack of capacity in a non-emergent situation, practitioners do not have carte blanche to perform all planned tests and procedures

INFORMED CONSENT

- Physicians are legally and ethically required to obtain informed consent of their patients before initiating treatment
- Consent must be knowing, intelligent, and voluntary
- Valid informed consent is premised on disclosure of appropriate information to a competent patient who is permitted to make a voluntary choice
- Capacity is a threshold question for being able to give informed consent
- When a patient cannot give informed consent, an alternate decision maker must be found
- Exceptions to informed consent apply narrowly:
  - Emergency exception: delivery of treatment without consent to a patient who is unconscious or in imminent danger of serious harm
  - Waiver: patient's right to waive disclosure of information (patient says he or she does not want to know)
  - Therapeutic privilege: doctor's decision to withhold information because telling the patient would cause psychological damage or render the patient ineffective in decision making. This is a very narrow exception that is not met when a patient would refuse treatment if information were given

REFERENCES

DELIRIUM

Breitbart W, Marotta R, Platt M, et. al. A Double-Blind Trial of Haloperidol, Chlorpromazine, and Lorazepam in the Treatment of Delirium in Hospitalized AIDS Patients. *AJP* 1996; 153(2):231–237.

Inouye SK. Delirium in Older Persons. *N Engl J Med* 2006;254:1157–1165.

Siddiqi N, House AO, Holmes, JD. Occurrence and outcome of delirium in medical inpatients: a systematic literature review. *Age and Ageing* 2006;35:350–364.

AGITATION

Allen MH, Currier GW. Use of restraints and pharmacotherapy in academic psychiatric emergency services. *Gen Hosp Psychiatry* 2004;26(1):42–49.

Marco CA, Vaughan J. Emergency management of agitation in schizophrenia. *Am J Emerg Med* 2005;23(6):767–776.

Marder SR. A review of agitation in mental illness: treatment guidelines and current therapies. *J Clin Psychiatry* 2006;67(suppl 10):13–21.

Moyer KE. A model of aggression with implications for research [proceedings]. *Psychopharmacol Bull* 1977;13(1):14–5.

Rosenbaum JF, Arana GW, Hyman SE, et al. *Handbook of Psychiatric Drug Therapy*, 5th ed. Philadelphia: Lippincott Williams & Wilkins; 2005:5–54.

Sachdev P, Kruk J. Restlessness: the anatomy of a neuropsychiatric symptom. *Aust N Z J Psychiatry* 1996;30:38–53.

Sachs GS. A review of agitation in mental illness: burden of illness and underlying pathology. *J Clin Psychiatry* 2006;67(suppl 10):5–12.

Teri L, Borson S, Kiyak HA, et al. Behavioral disturbance, cognitive dysfunction, and functional skill. Prevalence and relationship in Alzheimer's disease. *J Am Geriatr Soc* 1989;37(2):109–116.

CATATONIA

Fricchione GL, Huffman JC, Bush, G, et al. Catatonia, neuroleptic malignant syndrome, and serotonin syndrome. *Massachusetts General Hospital Comprehensive Clinical Psychiatry.* St. Louis: Mosby Elsevier; 2008:761–772.

Philbrick KL, Rummans TA. Malignant catatonia. *J Neuropsychiatry Clin Neurosci* 1994;6:1–13.

INTOXICATION, OVERDOSE, AND WITHDRAWAL

Eckardt MJ, Martin PR. Clinical assessment of cognition in alcoholism. *Alcohol Clin Exp Res* 1986;10:123.

Harding A, Halliday G, Caine D, et al. Degeneration of anterior thalamic nuclei differentiates alcoholics with amnesia. *Brain* 2000;123(pt 1):141–154.

Petit JR: *Handbook of Emergency Psychiatry.* Philadelphia: Lippincott Williams & Wilkins; 2004:123–138, 158–169, 220–232.

Repper-DeLisi J, Stern TA, Mitchell M, et al. Successful implementation of an alcohol-withdrawal pathway in a general hospital. *Psychosomatics* 2008;49:292–299.

Rosenbaum JF, Arana GW, Hyman SE, et al. *Handbook of Psychiatric Drug Therapy,* 5th ed. Philadelphia: Lippincott Williams & Wilkins; 2005:205–242.

Victor M, Adams RA, Collins GH. The Wernicke-Korsakoff syndrome and related disorders due to alcoholism and malnutrition, 2nd ed. Philadelphia: FA Davis Company; 1989.

SUICIDAL PATIENTS

Jacobs DG, Baldessarini RJ, Conwell Y et al. *Practice Guideline for the Assessment and Treatment of Patients with Suicidal Behaviors.* Arlington, VA: American Psychiatric Association; 2003.

Patterson WM, Dohn HH, Bird J, et al. Evaluation of Suicidal Patients: the SAD PERSONS Scale. *Psychosomatics* 1983;24:343–349.

Petit JR: *Handbook of Emergency Psychiatry.* Philadelphia: Lippincott Williams & Wilkins; 2004:189–203.

Sadock BJ, Sadock VA (eds). *Kaplan and Sadock's Synopsis of Psychiatry,* 9th ed. Philadelphia: Lippincott Williams & Wilkins; 2003:913–922.

HOMICIDAL PATIENTS

Sadock BJ, Sadock VA (eds). *Kaplan and Sadock's Synopsis of Psychiatry,* 9th ed. Philadelphia: Lippincott Williams & Wilkins; 2003:150–158.

NEUROLEPTIC MALIGNANT SYNDROME

Bhanushali MJ, Tuite PJ. The evaluation and management of patients with neuroleptic malignant syndrome. *Neurol Clin* 2004;22:394.

Nisijima Shioda K, Iwamura T. Neuroleptic malignant syndrome and serotonin syndrome. *Prog Brain Research* 2007;162:81–104.

Strawn JR, Keck PE Jr, Caroff SN. Neuroleptic malignant syndrome. *Am J Psychiatry* 2007;164:870–876.

Diagnostic and Statistical Manual of Mental Disorders, ed 4, rev text. Washington, DC: American Psychiatric Association; 2000:795–798.

SEROTONIN SYNDROME

Boyer EW, Shannon M. The serotonin syndrome. *N Engl J Med* 2005;352:1112–1120.

Nisijima Shioda K, Iwamura T, et al. Neuroleptic malignant syndrome and serotonin syndrome. *Prog Brain Research* 2007; 162:81–104.

LITHIUM TOXICITY

Delva NJ, Hawken ER. Preventing lithium intoxication: guide for physicians. *Can Fam Physician* 2001;47:1595–1600.

Freeman MP, Freeman SA. Lithium: clinical considerations in internal medicine. *Am J Med* 2006;119:478–481.

Rosenbaum JF, Arana GW, Hyman SE, et al. *Handbook of Psychiatric Drug Therapy*, 5th ed. Philadelphia: Lippincott Williams & Wilkins; 2005:147–149.

CAPACITY EVALUATION AND INFORMED CONSENT

Appelbaum PS. Assessment of patient's competence to consent to treatment. *N Engl J Med* 2007;357:1834–1840.

Brendel RW, Schouten R. Legal concerns in psychosomatic medicine. *Psychiatr Clin North Am* 2007;30(4):663–676.

Chapter 3

PSYCHIATRIC SYMPTOMS AND MANAGEMENT

Anxiety

Anxiety is common psychological state that often occurs in response to stress and is manifested by fear, worry, or nervousness. Such symptoms can be highly biologically adaptive if there is an actual threat to the individual but become maladaptive if they occur in the absence of a real threat and significantly impact functioning. The psychological symptoms

(*continued*)

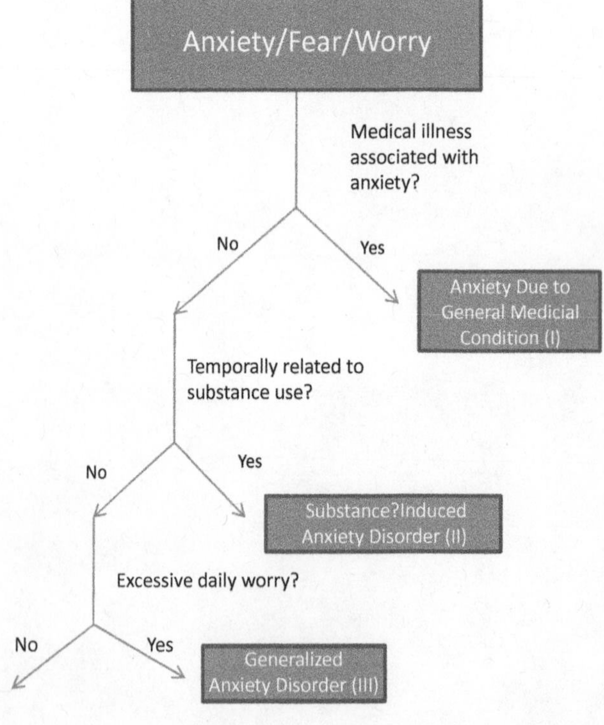

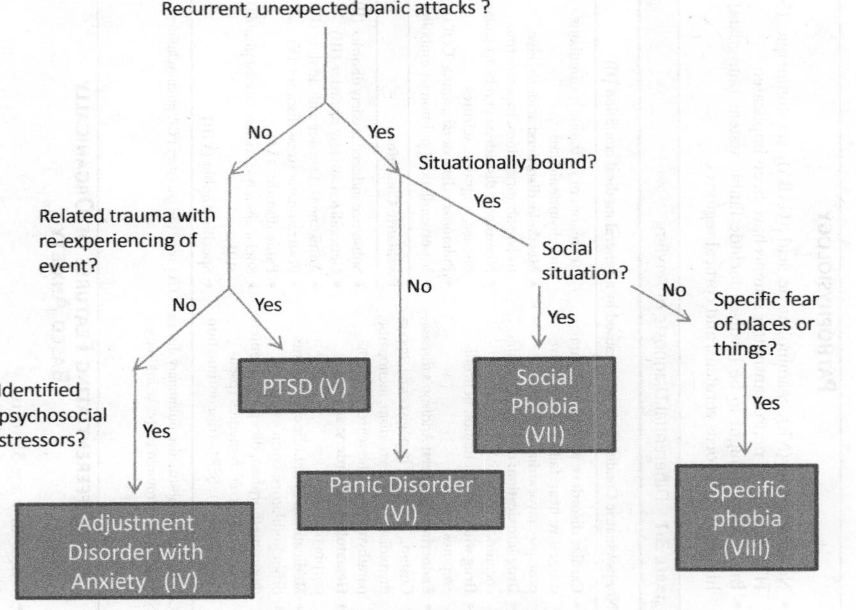

PTSD, posttraumatic stress disorder.

(*continued*)

are often accompanied by physical symptoms of autonomic arousal, including heart palpitations and sweating. Patients with many medical conditions also display similar symptoms, so it is crucial to rule out organic causes of anxiety.

PATHOPHYSIOLOGY

- Noradrenergic (NE), γ-aminobutyric acid (GABA), serotoninergic (5-HT), and other neurotransmitter systems have been implicated
- Brain areas thought to be involved include limbic system (amygdala), hippocampus, locus ceruleus, and cortical regions

TABLE 3-1 Differential Diagnosis of Anxiety

Nonpsychiatric Conditions (anxiety caused by a general medical condition [I])
• **Cardiac disorders:** angina, arrhythmia, congestive heart failure, mitral valve prolapse, myocardial infarction
• **Drug intoxication:** caffeine, cannabis, cocaine, PCP
• **Drug withdrawal:** ethanol, benzodiazepines
• **Endocrine disorders:** Addison's disease, Cushing's disease, hypoglycemia, hyperthyroidism, hypothyroidism, menopause, parathyroidism, pheochromocytoma
• **Hematologic disorders:** anemia, porphyria
• **Medications:** anticholinergic agents, bronchodilators, corticosteroids, dextromethorphan, diet pills (phentermine), OTC cold remedies (pseudoephedrine), SSRIs (discontinuation or treatment initiation), stimulants (methylphenidate)
• **Metabolic disorders:** acidosis, electrolyte abnormalities, hyperthermia
• **Neurologic disorders:** cerebrovascular disease, migraine, seizures
• **Pulmonary disorders:** asthma, COPD, hyperventilation, pulmonary embolus
Psychiatric Conditions
• Substance-induced anxiety disorder (II)
• Generalized anxiety disorder (III)
• Adjustment disorder with anxiety (IV)
• Posttraumatic stress disorder (V)
• Panic disorder (VI)
• Social anxiety disorder (social phobia) (VII)
• Specific phobia (VIII)

COPD, chronic obstructive pulmonary disease; OTC, over the counter; PCP, phencyclidine; SSRI, selective serotonin reuptake inhibitor.

DIFFERENTIATING FEATURES OF ORGANICALLY BASED ANXIETY

- Onset after age 35 years
- No personal or family history of anxiety disorder
- No childhood history of debilitating anxiety, separation anxiety, or phobias
- Lack of significant life events leading to or exacerbating anxiety symptoms
- Lack of avoidance behavior
- Poor response to anxiolytic medications

TABLE 3-2 Approach to the Evaluation of Anxiety

History with special attention to:
History of present illness: onset, symptoms, duration of current episode, other mood or psychotic symptoms, current substance use **Psychiatric history:** prior episodes (number of episodes, duration, average severity, time since last episode), other psychiatric disorders, substance use, medication trials
General Medical and Neurologic Examination
Psychiatric Mental Status Examination with special attention to:
Behavior (restless, fidgety), speech (increased rate), presence or absence of panic attacks
Laboratory Studies, Imaging, and Other Diagnostic Tools with special attention to:
If chest pain is present, persistent, and associated with other risk factors, consider EKG and further cardiac workup

EKG, electrocardiogram.

SUBSTANCE-INDUCED ANXIETY DISORDER (II)

- Prominent generalized anxiety, panic attacks, or obsessive–compulsive disorder (OCD) in the setting of substance intoxication or withdrawal
- Need confirmation from clinical history, laboratory results, or physical examination that either:
  - Anxiety developed during or within 1 month of substance intoxication or withdrawal
  - Substance use is etiologically related to anxiety symptoms
- Not occurring exclusively during delirium
- Diagnosis should only be made if anxiety exceeds symptoms usually seen in substance intoxication or withdrawal

GENERALIZED ANXIETY DISORDER (GAD) (III)

- The person has chronic, excessive worry or anxiety that occurs most days for at least 6 months
- It is associated with somatic symptoms, including fatigue, muscle tension, restlessness, sleep disturbance, difficulty concentrating, and irritability
- Anxiety is hard to control and causes significant impairment
- The person is seen as chronic "worrier" or "nervous person" by others around him or her

EPIDEMIOLOGY

- 3%–8% prevalence rate
- 2:1 female-to-male ratio
- 50%–90% have comorbid psychiatric illness

Adjustment Disorder with Anxiety (IV)

- Development of nervousness or worry occurring within 3 months of onset of psychosocial stressor
- Remits within 6 months after termination of stressor
- Not attributable to bereavement

Posttraumatic Stress Disorder (PTSD) (V)

- Intense fear, horror, and helplessness experienced after a traumatic event
- Trauma was such that patient directly witnessed, experienced, or was confronted with an event that involved actual or threatened death, injury, or threat to physical integrity
- Persistent reexperiencing of the event through distressing recollections, dreams, dissociative flashbacks, physiological reactivity, and psychological distress to stimulus cues of event
- Persistent avoidance of stimuli associated with the traumatic event and numbing of general responsiveness (e.g., detachment or sense of estrangement)
- Symptoms of hyperarousal are present, including:
  - Difficulty falling or staying asleep
  - Irritability or angry outbursts
  - Difficulty concentrating
  - Hypervigilance
  - Exaggerated startle response
- Symptoms present for more than 1 month (for symptoms <1 month, consider acute stress disorder)

Panic Disorder (PD) (VI)

- Recurrent, unexpected panic attacks
  - **Symptoms of panic attacks:** overwhelming anxiety or fear that comes on acutely (<10 min) and is accompanied by four or more of the symptoms below:
    - Chest pain
    - Palpitations
    - Derealization or depersonalization
    - Fear of dying, losing control, or losing one's mind
    - Paresthesias
    - Dizziness or lightheadedness
    - Shortness of breath
  - Many individuals may experience limited symptom attacks (e.g., only experiencing one or two of panic symptoms)

EPIDEMIOLOGY

- 3% of the general population
- Female > male
- Average age of onset: 24 years
- Potentially increased rate of suicidal ideation and attempts

- Attacks come on suddenly and peak within 10 minutes
- Accompanied by more than 1 month of more than one of following:
  - Anticipatory anxiety (so-called "fear of the fear")
  - Corresponding change in behavior (e.g., avoidance)
  - Worrying about consequences or outcomes of panic attacks
- May occur with or without agoraphobia
  - Agoraphobia
    - Anxiety caused by being in places or situations from which escape may be difficult or embarrassing or from which help may not be readily available in case of a panic attack
    - Typically involves clusters of situations outside the home, including being in a crowd; standing in line; being on a bridge; or traveling in a bus, train, or automobile
    - Situations are avoided or endured with marked distress or anxiety about having panic
- The first panic attack must occur unexpectedly (e.g., uncued)
- The person may become phobic of particular situation in which panic occurred, but anxiety is from fear of another panic attack. not the situation itself

SOCIAL ANXIETY DISORDER (SOCIAL PHOBIA) (VII)

- Excessive anxiety or fear triggered by social situations causing marked impairment
- Fear of being publicly scrutinized or humiliated
- Panic attacks are a common feature
- The patient recognizes that fear is excessive or irrational
- The phobic stimulus is avoided or lived through with significant anxiety
- Should specify if subtype "performance anxiety" is present

EPIDEMIOLOGY

- 3%–15% prevalence rate
- Onset peaks in adolescence
- Often comorbid with depression and substance abuse

SPECIFIC PHOBIA (VIII)

- Irrational, overwhelming fear of a specific situation or object
- Fear is recognized as irrational
- Avoidance of phobic stimulus is common
- Exposure to phobic stimulus can trigger panic attacks
- Causes marked impairment
- Types of phobias include animals (dogs), natural environment (heights), blood injection, situational (airplanes), and other (fear of choking)

EPIDEMIOLOGY

- 5%–10% of US population
- Most common psychiatric disorder among women; second among men
- Bimodal distribution of situational phobias: childhood and early adulthood

TREATMENT

Psychopharmacology Guidelines

- **Start slow:** patients with anxiety are very sensitive to somatic side effects

- **Selective serotonin reuptake inhibitors (SSRIs)** and **serotonin and norepinephrine reuptake inhibitors (SNRIs)** are **first-line agents** for most of the disorders
- Antidepressant doses used for depression may need to be higher
- Older agents such as **tricyclic antidepressants (TCAs)** and **monoamine oxidase inhibitors (MAOIs)** are effective but typically have more side effects
- TCAs are **not** effective for social anxiety disorder
- Benzodiazepine are efficacious, fast-acting, and generally well tolerated but have abuse liability
- There is a potential concern that benzodiazepines administered in aftermath of trauma may interfere with recovery after trauma
- Beta-blockers are sometimes used to **reduce autonomic arousal** in patients with panic attacks
- Beta-blockers are helpful in reducing the performance anxiety subtype but not the generalized subtype of social phobia

Psychotherapy Guidelines

- Anxiety disorders are effectively treated by many forms of psychotherapy, especially **cognitive behavior therapy (CBT)**
  - Cognitive restructuring: **restructures catastrophic thinking**
  - Relaxation training: **anxiety management** strategies
    - Slow breathing
    - Muscle relaxation
  - Behavioral exposure: repeatedly **exposing** the patient to **fearful stimuli** to extinguish the conditioned fear response
- Supportive therapy is particularly helpful for acute management immediately after the trauma of PTSD

Dementia

Definition

A chronic, progressive decline in cognitive abilities

Modified *Diagnostic and Statistical Manual of Mental Disorders IV (DSM-IV)*

Definition and Diagnostic Features

Cognitive deficits in areas listed in 1 and 2:

1. Problems with information recall or learning
2. One or more of the following problems with cognition:
   - Aphasia (problems with language)
   - Agnosia (difficulty recognizing objects)
   - Apraxia (difficulty executing voluntary movements without motor impairment)
   - Executive functioning problems (poor planning, abstract reasoning)
3. May also be associated with:
   - Poor judgment; disinhibition; hallucinations; delusions; anxiety, mood, or sleep disturbance

Dementia Diagnosis Categories and Representative Examples

TABLE 3-3 Dementia Diagnosis Categories and Representative Examples

Degenerative
- Alzheimer's dementia
- Dementia with Lewy bodies
- Frontotemporal dementia (e.g., Pick's disease)
- Parkinson's disease
- Huntington's disease
- Wilson's disease
- Progressive supranuclear palsy

Psychiatric
- Depression
- Schizophrenia

Vascular
- Vascular dementia
- Amyloid angiopathy

Obstructive
- Normal-pressure hydrocephalus

Traumatic
- Chronic subdural hematoma
- Dementia pugilistica

Neoplastic
- Malignant brain tumor
- Benign brain tumor
- Metastatic disease
- Paraneoplastic syndrome

Infectious
- HIV dementia
- Syphilis
- Creutzfeldt-Jakob disease

Demyelinating
- Multiple sclerosis

Autoimmune
- SLE

Drugs and Medications
- Anticholinergics
- Antihistamines
- Sedative–hypnotics

Substance Abuse
- Alcohol
- Narcotics
- Inhalants
- Prescription drug abuse

Toxins
- Arsenic
- Carbon monoxide
- Lead
- Mercury

HIV, human immunodeficiency virus; SLE, systemic lupus erythematosus

Adapted from Falk WE: The patient with memory problems or dementia. In Stern TA, Herman JB (eds). *The Massachusetts General Hospital Guide to Primary Care Psychiatry*, 2nd ed. New York: McGraw Hill; 2004:198. Reproduced with permission of the McGraw-Hill Companies.

Clinical Features of Delirium, Depression, and Alzheimer's Dementia

Alzheimer's dementia is the most common form of dementia. When evaluating a patient with known or suspected dementia, it is a priority to assess for delirium and treat the patient if necessary.

TABLE 3-4 Clinical Features of Delirium, Depression, and Alzheimer's Dementia

	Delirium	Depression	Alzheimer's Dementia
Onset	Abrupt	Relatively discrete	Insidious
Initial symptoms	Difficulty with attention and disturbed consciousness	Dysphoric mood or lack of pleasure	Memory deficits: verbal or spatial
Timeline	Fluctuating over days to weeks	Persistent; usually lasting months	Gradually progressive over years
Family history	Not contributory	May be positive for depression	May be positive for Alzheimer's dementia
Memory	Poor registration	Patchy or inconsistent loss of memory	Short-term memory worse than long-term memory
Subjective memory complaints	Absent	Present	Variable; usually absent
Example of language deficit	Difficulty attending to conversation or written tasks	Increased speech latency	Difficulty with naming objects
Affect	Often labile	Depressed or irritable	Can vary; may be neutral

Adapted from Falk WE: The patient with memory problems or dementia. In Stern TA, Herman JB (eds). *The Massachusetts General Hospital Guide to Primary Care Psychiatry,* 2nd ed. New York: McGraw Hill; 2004:198.

Behavioral Treatment Guidelines

- Safety of the patient and others takes priority. Use physical restraints or one-on-one supervision when necessary
- Consider behavioral interventions
  - Reorient to environment
  - Simplify communication
  - Reassure, distract, and redirect
- Identify if delirium is also present

Pharmacologic Treatment to Target Specific Symptoms

General Guidelines

- Minimize polypharmacy
- Identify and avoid drugs with cognitive side effects
- Assess for and treat comorbid medical problems, especially delirium

(*continued*)

TABLE 3-5 Approach to the Evaluation of Dementia

History with special attention to:
Source: family members, caregivers, patient (may be less reliable) **Presenting symptoms:** how difficulties first came to attention, deficits in recent memory suggests Alzheimer's disease; behavior change suggests frontotemporal dementia **Course:** gradual deterioration in Alzheimer's disease; stepwise deterioration in vascular dementia **Associated medical symptoms:** falls, incontinence, gait instability **Associated psychiatric symptoms:** hallucinations, paranoia, depressed or irritable mood, personality changes **Medical history:** stroke risk factors such as hypertension, diabetes **Psychiatric history:** mood disorder, substance abuse **Medications:** Include OTC medications; anticholinergics, psychiatric medications, narcotics may have cognitive effects **Family history:** Alzheimer's disease and frontotemporal dementia
General Medical and Neurologic Examination with special attention to:
Cardiovascular system, signs of infection, inflammation, and endocrine disorders **Cranial nerves, sensation, muscle tone and strength:** assess for focal abnormalities **Reflexes:** primitive reflexes (palmomental, glabellar, grasp, sucking) **Coordination and balance:** gait, position sense **Other:** asterixis, praxis, Luria maneuver
Psychiatric Mental Status Examination with special attention to:
Mood: depression may exacerbate or cause cognitive difficulty; irritability or elevated mood may be present in patients with mood disorders and dementia **Cognitive functioning:** attention, memory, orientation, language, executive functioning **Bedside and outpatient initial testing** • Folstein MMSE (published by Psychological Assessment Resources) • Montreal Cognitive Assessment (tests clock drawing, naming, word registration and recall, attention, abstraction, orientation) • Free test and interpretation guide available at www.mocatest.org
Laboratory Studies, Imaging, and Other Diagnostic Tools with special attention to:
First-line studies: Electrolytes, glucose, BUN or creatinine, CBC, liver function tests, thyroid function tests, lipids, B12 or folate levels, syphilis serology, urinalysis, CT scan (to rule out bleeding, NPH, stroke, tumor) **Second-line studies, if indicated:** brain MRI (especially if neurologic examination is abnormal), EEG (assess for seizure, metabolic encephalopathy), lumbar puncture (assess for infection, cancer, vasculitis), HIV testing, autoimmune disorder screening tests, drug levels, heavy metal screening, ECG, CXR **Testing referral** may be indicated if initial screening is abnormal and there are questions regarding diagnosis or functional ability

BUN, blood urea nitrogen; CBC, complete blood count; CT, computed tomography; CXR, chest radiography; ECG, electrocardiography; EEG, electroencephalography; HIV, human immunodeficiency virus; MMSE, Mini-Mental Status Examination; MRI, magnetic resonance imaging; NPH, normal-pressure hydrocephalus; OTC, over the counter.

TABLE 3-6 Dementia Subtypes

	Alzheimer's Disease	Vascular Dementia	Lewy Body Dementia	Frontotemporal Dementia (e.g., Pick's Disease)	Normal-Pressure Hydrocephalus
Epidemiology	Most common dementia; age >70 years	Second most common; associated with vascular risk factors	Age >70 years; associated with Parkinson's disease	Most common early-onset dementia; appears in 50s and 60s	Occurs after trauma, infection, or hemorrhage rather than being idiopathic
Initial symptoms	Short-term memory loss	Apathy, gait problems, memory loss	Parkinsonism (rigidity, bradykinesia), sleep disturbance, visual hallucinations	Personality changes (apathy, disinhibition)	Triad of shuffling gait, urinary incontinence, and cognitive impairment
Prominent cognitive symptoms	Progressive memory impairment, disorientation, aphasia, apraxia, agnosia	Visuospatial deficits, slowed processing, impaired memory retrieval	Episodic fluctuations in arousal or alertness	Disinhibition, aphasia if left sided; memory relatively preserved	Slowed verbal responses
Noncognitive symptoms	Depression, apathy, delusions, hostility	Depression, psychosis	VH or illusions, delusions (misidentification or Capgras), autonomic dysfunction, falls or postural instability	Stereotyped motor behaviors, compulsions, hyperorality, antisocial personality, impulsivity (gambling, sexual or verbal disinhibition)	Apathy, depression

Neuropsychological deficits	Short-term memory, attention, orientation	Visuospatial deficits, executive dysfunction	Visuospatial deficits, executive dysfunction	Executive dysfunction, memory and visuospatial preserved	Executive dysfunction
Imaging	Generalized atrophy (parietal, temporal, hippocampal)	Subcortical white matter	Subtle parietal or occipital atrophy	Frontotemporal atrophy (frontal or temporal subvariants)	Enlarged ventricles
Neuropathology	β-Amyloid plaques, neurofibrillary tangles	Microvascular ischemic changes	α-Synuclein, Lewy bodies	Tau, ubiquitin	
Treatment	Cholinesterase inhibitors; memantine for moderate to severe cases	Manage vascular risk factors: smoking, HTN, hyperlipidemia; cholinesterase inhibitors	Cholinesterase inhibitors; avoid typical neuroleptics because they induce EPS; quetiapine for psychosis	SSRIs, antipsychotics; cholinesterase inhibitors have limited benefit	Ventriculoperitoneal shunt

EPS, extrapyramidal side effects; HTN, hypertension; SSRI, selective serotonin reuptake inhibitor; VH, visual hallucinations.

(continued)

- Start with low doses (one quarter to one half that for normal adults) and increase slowly while monitoring for side effects
- Older patients may be more sensitive to medication side effects such as sedation, orthostatic hypotension, anticholinergic side effects, and extrapyramidal side effects (EPS)
- No pharmacologic treatment exists for wandering behavior

TABLE 3-7 Suggested Pharmacologic and Somatic Treatments for Symptoms Occurring with Dementia

Symptom	Treatment
Cognitive symptoms	**Cognitive enhancers** (e.g., donepezil, galantamine, rivastigmine, memantine): generally not helpful in the acute setting but may have long-term beneficial effects on behavior and mood
Depression	**SSRIs:** avoid those with greater anticholinergic side effects (e.g., paroxetine) **Other antidepressants:** mirtazapine, bupropion **Stimulants:** methylphenidate • For poor energy or motivation • Use with caution in patients with cardiac disease **MAOIs or ECT:** for severe, treatment-refractory depression
Hallucinations, paranoia, delusions	**Atypical antipsychotics** **Typical antipsychotics:** generally avoid agents with greater anticholinergic effect (e.g., thioridazine)
Agitation (restlessness, verbal outbursts, physical aggression)	**Atypical antipsychotics** **Typical antipsychotics:** generally avoid agents with greater anticholinergic effect (e.g., thioridazine) **Benzodiazepines:** caution: risk of disinhibition, worsened cognition **Other agents:** trazodone, propanol, valproic acid

ECT, electroconvulsive therapy; MAOI, monoamine oxidase inhibitor; SSRI, selective serotonin reuptake inhibitor.

Guidelines Regarding Antipsychotic Use

- Hallucinations, paranoia, and delusions may not require treatment unless they are causing great distress to the patient or potential harm to others
- When using atypical antipsychotics, consider the risk–benefit ratio for each patient and talk with patients and their families about the Food and Drug Administration (FDA) black box warning regarding a possible increased risk of death from medication use
- Patients with dementia with Lewy bodies (which often co-occurs with Alzheimer's dementia) are often very sensitive to antipsychotics. (Recall that antipsychotics may cause akathisia and agitation)

Depression

Depression is a common symptom, with up to 25% of the US population experiencing a depressive episode at some point during their lives. A recent report from the Centers for Disease Control and Prevention's National Center for Health Statistics shows that in any 2-week period, more than one in 20 Americans are depressed. Given its prevalence and morbidity, depression deserves due attention and treatment.

TABLE 3-8 Differential Diagnosis of Depression

Nonpsychiatric Conditions	Psychiatric Conditions
• Thyroid disorders • Adrenal disorders • Metabolic disturbances (e.g., hypercalcemia, hyponatremia) • Diabetes mellitus • Medication-induced (beta-blockers, CCBs, barbiturates, cholinergic medications, corticosteroids, estrogens) • Nutritional deficiencies (vitamin B12, folate, pellagra) • Malignancy • Neurologic disease (CVA, subdural hematoma, MS, tumor)	• Major depressive episode • Major depressive disorder • Dysthymia • Adjustment disorder with depressed mood • Bipolar disorder • Schizoaffective disorder • Bereavement • Substance abuse (including alcohol or withdrawal from stimulants)

CCB, calcium channel blockers; CVA, cerebrovascular accident; MS, multiple sclerosis.

Major Depressive Episode (MDE)

- MDE is defined by five or more of the following symptoms, one of which must be depressed mood or anhedonia. All symptoms must occur in the same 2-week period, be present a minimum of most of the day on most days, and result in clinically significant social, occupation, or interpersonal impairment
  - Depressed mood
  - Profound loss of interest or pleasure in all or almost all activities (anhedonia)
  - Profound increase (atypical feature) or decrease in appetite
  - Insomnia or hypersomnia (atypical feature)
  - Objective psychomotor hyperactivity or retardation
  - Decreased energy
  - Indecisiveness or decreased concentration
  - Worthlessness or guilt
  - Recurrent thoughts of death, recurrent suicidal ideation (SI) without a plan, SI with a plan, or suicide attempt (SA)

"SIGECAPS"
Sleep (increased or decreased) **I**nterest (anhedonia)
Guilt (feeling worthless or hopeless)
Energy (decreased)
Concentration (decreased)
Appetite (increased or decreased)
Psychomotor retardation or agitation
Suicidal ideation

TABLE 3-9 Approach to the Evaluation of Depression

History with special attention to:	**Psychiatric Mental Status Examination** with special attention to:
Common chief complaints: • Reduced energy or fatigue (occurs in >90% of patients with MDD) • Impairment at work or school • Social isolation • Decreased motivation • Difficulties with sleep, particularly with early morning waking • Anxiety • Disturbances of sexual functioning • Problems with concentration or thinking and memory **Psychiatric history:** history of suicidal thoughts or attempts (those with prior hospitalization for SI or SA have a greater lifetime risk of completed suicide) **Social history:** screen for social isolation	• General appearance: psychomotor retardation or agitation, decreased eye contact, inadequate hygiene • Mood: down, depressed (although patient may deny feeling depressed), irritable, anxious, labile • Affect: restricted, blunted • Thought process: slowed • Thought content: may include delusions • Perceptions: psychotic hallucinations • Speech: slowed with flattened tone or volume
General Medical and Neurologic Examination with special attention to:	**Laboratory Studies, Imaging, and Other Diagnostic Tools** with special attention to:
Signs of intoxication or withdrawal; thyroid abnormalities (sweating, tachycardia, tremor, cold intolerance, weight gain); increased ICP (ocular abnormalities)	**First-line studies:** toxicology screen, TSH, CBC, chemistry panel 7, UA **Second-line studies, if indicated:** cortisol, HIV, liver function tests, B12, head imaging

CBC, complete blood count; HIV, human immunodeficiency virus; ICP, intracranial pressure MDD, major depressive disorder; SA, suicide attempt; SI, suicidal ideation; TSH, thyroid-stimulating hormone; UA, urinalysis.

MAJOR DEPRESSIVE DISORDER (MDD)

- Presence of at least one depressive episode
- Rule out a history of manic, mixed, or hypomanic episodes; psychotic disorder; and delusional disorder
- Modifiers include:
  - For active MDE: mild, moderate, severe with or without psychotic, melancholic, atypical, or postpartum features
  - If full criteria for MDE are not present: partial vs. full remission with or without psychotic, melancholic, atypical, or postpartum features
- Two thirds of people with MDE contemplate suicide; 10% to 15% commit suicide
- There is a 50% recurrence rate after the first episode, a 70% recurrence rate after the second episode, and a 90% recurrence after the third episode

EPIDEMIOLOGY

- Lifetime risk: women: 20%–25%; men 7%–12%
- No socioeconomic or racial correlation
- Increased in single people
- Circumstances that may increase risk: being single, living in a rural area, divorced, losing a parent before age 11 years, experiencing the death of spouse, unemployment

Dysthymia

- Defined by depressed mood most of the day for more days than not for 2 years with symptom-free periods not exceeding 2 months during the 2-year period
- While the patient is depressed, two of the following must be present:
  - Increased or decreased appetite
  - Insomnia or hypersomnia
  - Fatigue or low energy
  - Low self-esteem
  - Indecisiveness or decreased concentration
  - Hopelessness

Adjustment Disorder with Depressed Mood

- Depression resulting in significant clinical impairment but not meeting the criteria for major depression
- Occurs within 3 months of a stressful life event and does not persist longer than 6 months after termination of the stressor

Bereavement

- Depressive symptoms occurring within 2 months of the death of a loved one are considered normal grief
- Certain symptoms after the death may be associated with MDD:
  - Guilt (not including guilt regarding actions taken or not taken by survivor at the time of death)
  - Thoughts of death (not including patient feeling he or she would be better off dead or should have died with the deceased person)
  - Morbid preoccupation with worthlessness
  - Marked psychomotor retardation
  - Substantial, prolonged functional impairment
  - Hallucinations (not including transient seeing or hearing of the deceased person)

Treatment of Depression

- There is a 40% remission rate with an adequate single trial with an antidepressant; the majority of the rest of patients show some improvement, but 15% to 30% of patients do not improve after a single adequate trial
- The most common reasons for failure are inadequate dosing and inadequate duration
- Suggested pharmacotherapy guidelines:
  - No single antidepressant is universally accepted as more effective than another
  - Therapy should be chosen based on side effects, drug interactions, dosing schedule, discontinuation symptoms, cost of treatment, and history of effective response (including history of response in a first-degree relative)

- Before declaring treatment failure, ensure maximum titration and minimum of 4 to 6 weeks of treatment after achieving the maximum dose (full response is gauged at 8–12 weeks)
- Duration of treatment for depression maintenance:
  - Single episode: treat for a minimum of 6 months after resolution of symptoms or for the length of previous depressive episode, whichever is longer
  - Multiple episodes: indefinite maintenance
- Addressing inadequate treatment response (treatment failure or partial response, defined as a 20% to 25% reduction in depressive symptoms):
  - Ensure proper dosing and duration of medication
  - Consider the accuracy of the diagnosis
  - If there is no response, switch the class of medication
  - If there is a less than desired response: augmentation with lithium or thyroid hormone (T3)

TABLE 3-10 Suggested Treatment by Depressive Subtype

Subtype	Treatment
Atypical depression (predominantly depressed mood, hyperphagia, and hypersomnia)	MAOI, SSRI, bupropion, augmentation with D2 or D3 antagonist (pramipexole or ropinirole)
Melancholic (predominant anhedonia, early morning waking, excessive guilt, reduced appetite or weight loss, psychomotor retardation and agitation)	SNRI, TCA
Irritability or anger attacks	SSRI
Seasonal affective type (recurring depression during winter months, with decreased activity, lethargy, increased eating, increased sleep, social isolation, decreased sex drive)	Light therapy: 10 K lux for 30 minutes in the morning and the evening
Depression with psychosis	Increased risk of SI, antidepressant alone: 30%–50% response vs. 70%–80% with addition of antipsychotic; ECT if addition of antipsychotic fails or rapid treatment is necessary
Multiple treatment failures, severe symptoms, or concurrent pregnancy	ECT
Depression with concurrent panic disorder	TCA or SSRI
Depression with concurrent substance abuse	Abstinence (may treat depression as well)

ECT, electroconvulsive therapy; MAOI, monoamine oxidase inhibitor; SI, suicidal ideation; SNRI, serotonin and norepinephrine reuptake inhibitor; SSRI, selective serotonin reuptake inhibitor; TCA, tricyclic antidepressant.

Disordered Eating Behaviors

Both underweight and overweight patients should be evaluated for eating disorders. Given the high morbidity and mortality associated with eating disorders, it is extremely important to identify and treat these patients expediently.

TABLE 3-11 Differential Diagnosis of Disordered Eating Behaviors

Nonpsychiatric Conditions
Weight loss: thyroid disease, malignancy, infectious diseases (including HIV), GI absorptive diseases (i.e., celiac disease), other causes of amenorrhea (including pregnancy, PCOS, pituitary disease or Sheehan's syndrome, ovarian failure or menopause), epileptic-equivalent seizures, malignancies, diabetes mellitus, HIV **Weight gain:** Cushing's syndrome, steroids, medication side effects, lifestyle (overeating, lack of exercise), Klein-Levin syndrome (hypersomnia or hyperphagia), Kluver-Bucy syndrome (hyperorality or hypersexuality)
Psychiatric
• Anorexia nervosa (AN) • Bulimia nervosa (BN) • Eating disorder NOS • Binge eating disorder • Major depression (frequently associated with decreased appetite and weight changes) • Somatization disorder (GI symptoms such as nausea and vomiting; menstrual difficulties) • Schizophrenia • Body dysmorphic disorder

GI, gastrointestinal; HIV, human immunodeficiency virus; NOS, not otherwise specified; PCOS, polycystic ovary syndrome.

Epidemiology and Definitions of Eating Disorders

Anorexia Nervosa (AN)

- Significantly low weight (≥15% below expected body weight) in combination with resistance to weight gain, often motivated by excessive concern with thinness or control overeating
- Low weight is maintained by dietary restriction but is frequently accompanied by purging and exercise (see Bulimia nervosa)
- Lifetime prevalence: 0.9% in women; 0.3% in men

Bulimia Nervosa (BN)

- Characterized by regular episodes of binge eating followed by a variety of purging, exercise, and dietary behaviors to prevent weight gain
- Lifetime prevalence: 1.0%–1.5% in women (*continued*)

TABLE 3-12 Approach to the Evaluation of Disordered Eating

History with special attention to:
History of present illness: evaluate motivation for change, past response to therapy, nutritional compromise impacting psychosocial treatment, requirements for level of care **Psychiatric history:** high comorbidity with affective disorders, anxiety disorder, OCD, personality disorders **Medical history:** menstrual dysfunction (amenorrhea, irregular menstruation), GI dysfunction (slowed motility, nausea, bloating) **Family history:** more prevalent among patients with a first-degree relative with an eating disorder or alcoholism **Social history:** risk factors include a history of dieting and participating in sports in which leanness is emphasized (ballet, running, wrestling) or in which scoring is subjective (skating, gymnastics) **Review of systems:** evaluate for hair loss, dry skin, headache, concentration, sleep issues, cold intolerance, fatigue, weakness, fainting, dizziness, irregular heart beat, dyspepsia, diarrhea, constipation, menses, muscle cramps, nocturia
General Medical and Neurologic Examination with special attention to:
Evidence of undernutrition, low weight, and purging, including growth delay, dental enamel erosion, enlarged parotid glands, cognitive changes, weight, height, vital signs (including orthostatics) **Calculate** BMI or percentage of expected body weight based on weight, height, gender, and stage of development • Ensure that weight is taken before hydration ("dry weight") • Rough guideline: 100 lb for 5′ and 5 lb for each additional inch for women; 106 lb for 5′ and 6 lb for each additional inch for men
Psychiatric Mental Status Examination with special attention to:
Mental status changes that could be attributed to significant medical compromise such as electrolyte disturbance
Laboratory Studies, Imaging, and Other Diagnostic Tools with special attention to:
First-line studies: ECG (QTc prolongation), endocrine laboratory studies (↓LH, ↓FSH, ↑cortisol, ↑GH), electrolytes (hypokalemia, metabolic alkalosis), blood glucose, CBC, renal function, TSH **Second-line studies, if indicated:** bone densitometry (osteopenia, osteoporosis)

BMI, body mass index; CBC, complete blood count; ECG, electrocardiography; FSH, follicle-stimulating hormone; GH, growth hormone; GI, gastrointestinal; LH, luteinizing hormone; OCD, obsessive–compulsive disorder; TSH, thyroid-stimulating hormone.

(*continued*)

Eating Disorder Not Otherwise Specified (NOS)

- Aberrant eating patterns and weight management habits not meeting criteria for AN or BN
- The most common presentation of eating disorders
- Occurs in 3% to 5% of women age 15 to 30 years

Binge Eating Disorder (BED)

- Episodic binge eating without purging, exercise, and dietary behaviors to prevent weight gain
- Eating not linked to cues (social, hunger, satiety) that conventionally drive eating
- Episodes may be associated with distress and other negative affect
- At least three of the following must be present:
  - Eating more rapidly than normal
  - Eating until feeling uncomfortably full
  - Eating large amounts of food when not feeling hungry
  - Eating alone because of embarrassment of how much one is eating
  - Feeling disgusted with oneself, depressed, or guilty of overeating
- Lifetime prevalence: 3.5% in women; 2% in men

Treatment

Medical

- Evaluate the patient's medical and nutritional compromise
- Treat the medical sequelae of undernutrition, purging behaviors, and obesity
- Watch for refeeding syndrome caused by low phosphorous (gastric bloating, congestive heart failure (CHF), edema; can lead to respiratory failure, coma, seizures, or death)
- Surveillance for and treatment of common and life-threatening complications, such as medical sequela of BN (tooth enamel decay, esophagitis, blistered knuckles) or emergencies such as arrhythmias or hematemesis
- Management of obesity-related complications in patients with BED (diabetes, sleep apnea, dyslipidemia, cardiovascular disease)

Nutritional

- Determine energy and micronutrient deficits and protocol for nutritional rehabilitation
- The patient may safely gain 0.5 to 2.0 lb per week as an outpatient or up to 3 to 4 lb as an inpatient
- Provide vitamin supplementation

Psychiatric and Psychosocial

- Section 12 criteria for admission to inpatient psychiatric facility after medical stabilization: the patient must demonstrate him- or herself to be unable to care for him- or herself, as evidenced by weight below 75% of ideal body weight, electrolyte disturbance (K <3.2), electrocardiographic changes, abnormal vital signs (i.e., bradycardia, low blood pressure, significant orthostatic changes, hypothermia), or indications of suicidality
- Patients under 20% of expected weight for their height should be enrolled in inpatient programs

- Treatment initially supports nutritional goals and medical and psychiatric stabilization
  - Family therapy is the treatment of choice for adolescents with AN
  - CBT and interpersonal therapy (IPT) have been demonstrated effective for BN

Pharmacologic

GENERAL GUIDELINES

- Treat common comorbid psychiatric conditions, such as depression and anxiety
- Medications that modify appetite: mirtazapine: increase appetite; topiramate: decrease appetite; Meridia: appetite suppressant
- Monitor for potential weight gain as a medication side effect (i.e., with atypical antipsychotics)

ANTIDEPRESSANTS

- There are no FDA-approved medications for the treatment of AN
- Fluoxetine is FDA approved for treatment of BN (higher dosing, 60–80 mg)
- Antidepressant use should not be initiated until weight gain has been achieved because side effects can be more severe in malnourished patients
- Bupropion is contraindicated in patients with BN because of an increased risk of seizures

ANTIPSYCHOTICS

- Some data suggest that atypical antipsychotics may have benefits for some AN patients, but this use is off label and has no established efficacy
- Use with caution because of the risk for idiopathic and hypokalemia-related QT prolongation

OTHER

- Antiepileptics have shown some effectiveness anecdotally in patients with BED
- Zinc (50–100 mg) has been shown to more rapidly improve weight restoration in patients with AN

Dissociation

Dissociation is a process by which mental contents (cognitions, emotions, sensations, behaviors) become segregated from one another. This process exists along a continuum from normative to pathological (Steinberg, 2000).

During exposure to traumatic stress, dissociation may serve an adaptive function by buffering the impact of overwhelming experience. However, with repeated exposures, dissociation may become conditioned as a primary defense and occur chronically in response to reminders of the original traumatic event or even to relatively minor stressors of everyday living (Howell, 2005).

Types of Dissociative Experiences

Normative

- Daydreaming
- Becoming absorbed in a movie or a book
- Meditation
- "Highway hypnosis" (e.g., being briefly lost in a trance while driving)
- Fantasy
- Formal or self-induced hypnotic state

Pathological

- **Numbing:** feeling detached from one's emotions
- **Flashback:** intrusive immersion in sensory components of a past traumatic experience
- **Depersonalization:** feeling detached from one's self or looking at one's self as an outsider would
- **Derealization:** feeling detached from one's environment or a sense that the environment is unreal or foreign
- **Amnesia:** inability to account for a specific and significant block of time that has passed
- **Identity confusion:** feeling uncertain, puzzled, or conflicted about who one is
- **Identity alteration:** shifting of one's role or identity, accompanied by changes in behavior (*continued*)

TABLE 3-13 Differential Diagnosis of Dissociative Experiences

Nonpsychiatric Conditions	
Depersonalization: hypoglycemia, hypothyroidism, migraine, temporal lobe epilepsy or lesion, nondominant parietal lobe lesion, SLE, hypnogogic or hypnopompic phenomena **Derealization:** temporal lobe epilepsy or lesion, hypnogogic or -pompic phenomena **Amnesia:** Cerebral anoxia, cerebral tumor, head trauma, herpes encephalitis, hippocampal infarction, transient global amnesia, Wernicke-Korsakoff syndrome	
Psychiatric Conditions	
• Acute stress disorder • PTSD • Dissociative amnesia • Dissociative fugue	• Depersonalization disorder • Dissociative identity disorder • Dissociative disorder NOS

NOS, not otherwise specified; PTSD, posttraumatic stress disorder; SLE, systemic lupus erythematosus.

TABLE 3-14 Approach to the Evaluation of Dissociation

History with special attention to:

Screening questions for dissociative disorders (Lowenstein, 1991):
- **Absorption:** "Do you ever become preoccupied with daydreams inside your head for hours at a time?"
- **Numbing:** "Do you ever feel detached from your feelings or emotions?"
- **Flashbacks:** "Do you ever experience a frightening event from the past with such intensity that you lose track of where you are in the present? Do you hear it, see it, and smell it?"
- **Depersonalization:** "Do you ever feel as if your body is unreal or you are outside your body observing yourself?"
- **Derealization:** "Do you ever feel as if your surroundings are foggy or unreal?"
- **Amnesia:** "Do you have gaps in the continuity of your memory for childhood?" and "Do you have blank spells or lose time?"
- **Identity alteration:** "Do you hear voices inside your head talking with each other and to you?" and "Do you feel like there is more than one person or part inside of you?"

Social history: screen for trauma

General Medical and Neurologic examination

Psychiatric Mental Status Examination

Laboratory Studies, Imaging, and Other Diagnostic Tools with special attention to:

Use the nonpsychiatric differential above and use laboratory, neuroimaging, EEG, and sleep study testing as indicated

EEG, electroencephalography.

(continued)

Acute Stress Disorder (ASD)

- Requires experience of a traumatic event, occurrence of three to five dissociative symptoms, one reexperiencing symptoms, and marked avoidance and arousal at the time of or shortly after the event
- Occurs within 1 month of the traumatic event and persists for at least 2 days
- Recognizes dissociative symptoms as frequent sequelae to traumatic exposure

Posttraumatic Stress Disorder (PTSD)

- See page 56 for more information
- Requires experience of a traumatic stressor, occurrence of one reexperiencing symptom, three avoidance symptoms, and two arousal symptoms for duration of more than 1 month after the event
- Does not require dissociative symptoms for diagnosis; however, several dissociative symptoms fall under PTSD diagnostic criteria, including flashbacks, numbing, detachment, restricted affect or absence of emotional responsiveness, and amnesia

Dissociative Amnesia

- One or multiple episodes of memory loss typified by inability to recall important personal information (e.g., one's identity or significant elements of one's past)
- Occasionally seen in adult-onset traumatic events
- The unrecalled personal information is often of a stressful or traumatic nature
- Occurs outside the context of a diagnosed traumatic stress disorder, other dissociative disorder, or somatization disorder

Dissociative Fugue

- Sudden, unexpected travel away from one's home or workplace associated with memory loss and confusion about one's personal identity
- Rarely occurs outside the context of dissociative identity disorder

Depersonalization Disorder

- Persistent and recurrent episodes of feeling detached from one's self, body, thoughts, and feelings
- Reality testing is normal
- Common immediate precipitants of the disorder are severe stress, depression, panic, marijuana ingestion, and hallucinogen ingestion
- Must occur outside the context of dissociative identity disorder
- Not necessarily associated with trauma and may be caused by high innate dissociative capacity

Dissociative Identity Disorder (DID)

- Existence of two or more distinct and coherent identities or self-states
- At least two self-states assume control of one's thought processes and behavior
- Chronic inability to recall important personal information about one's past
- Typical symptomatology may include hearing voices (generally inside the head), gaps in memory, and being told or finding evidence of unremembered behaviors

Dissociative Disorder Not Otherwise Specified (DDNOS)

- Primary symptom is dissociation, but the presentation does not meet full criteria for another dissociative disorder
- Atypical DID (e.g., dissociative identities without memory loss)
- Derealization that occurs without depersonalization
- Sequela of prolonged thought coercion practices (e.g., brainwashing)
- Cross-cultural phenomena: purposeful induction of a trance or possession state

Treatment of Acute Traumatic Stress and Dissociative Reactions

General Guidelines

- The eventual, definitive treatment of trauma-spectrum disorders involves a gradual working through of the underlying traumatic experience(s) within the context of a consistent and supportive therapeutic relationship
- However, in the acute setting, the primary treatment aim is to work with the patient to establish a sense of safety by containing posttraumatic and dissociative symptoms

Behavioral Interventions

- Help the patient feel safe and oriented to the present
  - Move the patient to a quiet, well-lit room
  - Ask the patient to maintain eye contact
  - Tell the patient in a firm, reassuring voice that you are there to help and will assist him or her to stay in the present
- Use **"grounding techniques"** to reduce preoccupation with trauma, flashbacks, and dissociative symptoms
  - Ask the patient to look around and focus objects in the room, naming them out loud
  - Ask the patient to hold a familiar object with a strong sensation, such as a piece of ice, and describe what he or she feels
  - Other interventions involving the different senses include listening to music; singing; or smelling strong, pleasant scents such as oranges or coffee

Psychopharmacology

- Adjunctive
- Likely treating the hyperarousal symptoms associated with PTSD
- **Anxiolytics** may be helpful in treating associated anxiety (e.g., lorazepam 1–2 mg, repeated as needed)
- **Neuroleptics**, particularly atypicals, may be helpful in treating associated chronic anxiety, insomnia, and irritability (e.g., risperidone 0.5–1.0 mg; quetiapine 25–50 mg)

Mania

Mania is a severe psychiatric symptom affecting approximately 1% of the population and characterized by elevated, expansive, or irritable mood. Patients may derive pleasure during episodes of mania; however, their actions during these episodes often have negative financial, personal, and medical consequences. Mania therefore must be treated promptly and effectively, often with hospitalization and pharmacologic interventions.

TYPES OF MANIC EPISODES

- **Manic Episode**
  - A period of abnormally and continually irritable, expansive or elevated mood which lasts at least one week. If hospitalization is necessary, it is automatically considered mania
  - At least three of the following symptoms must be present (or at least four if mood is only irritable) of the following:
    - Grandiosity
    - Decreased need for sleep
    - Excessive or pressured speech
    - Racing thoughts (subjective) or flight of ideas (objective)
    - Distractibility
    - Increased goal-directed activity
    - Impulsivity or excessive involvement in pleasurable or dangerous activities
  - The episode causes a marked impairment of functioning and is not caused by a substance, medication, or other medical condition
- **Hypomanic Episode**
  - A period of abnormally and continually irritable, expansive, or elevated mood which lasts throughout at least four days and is clearly not depressed, and during which the patient has suffered from at least three manic symptoms (see above)
  - The change in mood is observable by others, does **not** impair functioning, does not involve psychotic features, and is not caused by a substance, medication, or other medical condition
- **Mixed Episode**
  - The patient meets criteria for both a major depressive episode (except for duration) and a manic episode nearly every day for at least one week
  - The episode causes a marked impairment of functioning and is not caused by a substance, medication, or other medical condition

"DIGFAST"

Distractibility
Impulsivity/excessive pleasure
Grandiosity
Flight of ideas
Activity (increased)
Sleep (decreased need)
Talkativeness (pressured speech)

EPIDEMIOLOGY

- Peak age of onset: 15–24 years
- Lifetime prevalence: 0.8%
- 90% of patients who suffer one manic episode will have another and 10%–15% of patients will have >10 manic episodes.

PATHOPHYSIOLOGY

- Manic patients have lower levels of choline (precursor to acetylcholine) and serotonin metabolites
- Possible involvement of the prefrontal-subcortical-limbic system circuitry
- Hypothalamic-pituitary-thyroid axis abnormalities more common in bipolar patients.
- 40%–70% lifetime risk of bipolar disorder in monozygotic twins (5%–10% in other 1st-degree relatives)

Treatment (Hirschfeld et al., 2002)

- Acute mania
  - First-line
    - Severe: lithium plus atypical antipsychotic OR valproate plus atypical antipsychotic
    - Less severe: monotherapy (lithium, valproate, or atypical antipsychotic)

- Alternatives: carbamazepine, oxcarbazepine
- If first-line therapy fails:
  - Add a second first-line agent
  - Add carbamazepine
  - Add/change antipsychotic

TABLE 3-15 Differential Diagnosis

Non-psychiatric Conditions	**Neurological disorders** Strokes, Huntington's disease, multiple sclerosis, complex partial seizures, brain tumors **Infectious diseases** HIV, tertiary syphilis **Endocrine disorders** Thyrotoxicosis **Rheumatic disorders** Systemic lupus erythematosus (SLE) **Substance-induced** Cocaine, amphetamines, alcohol, hallucinogens, PCP, antidepressants, dopamine agonists, decongestants, steroids, immunosuppressants, certain chemotherapeutic agents
Psychiatric Conditions	**Bipolar I disorder** At least one manic or mixed episode; men = women **Bipolar II disorder** At least one major depressive episode and at least one hypomanic episode WITHOUT a manic or mixed episode; men < women **Cyclothymic disorder** Numerous hypomanic episodes and periods with depressive symptoms that do NOT meet criteria for a major depressive episode and last at least two years without being symptom-free for more than two months at a time. **Schizoaffective disorder** A major depressive, manic, or mixed episode concurrent with symptoms of schizophrenia and presence of psychotic symptoms for at least 2 weeks in absence of mood symptoms.

TABLE 3-16 Mood Disorders and the Episodes Required for Diagnosis

	Manic	Hypomanic	Depressive	Dysthymic
MDD			X	+/−
Bipolar I D/O	X	+/−	+/−	+/−
Bipolar II D/O		X	X	+/−
Dysthymic D/O				X
Cyclothymic D/O		X		X

  - Treatment-refractory: clozapine or ECT
  - Discontinue antidepressants
- Maintenance therapy
  - First-line: lithium, olazapine, aripiprazole, quetiapine, or valproate
  - Alternatives: lamotrigine, carbamazepine
  - If acute episode of mania responded to a particular medication, that drug may be continued

TABLE 3-17 Approach to the Evaluation for Mania

History with special attention to:
History of Present Illness: Include onset, symptoms, duration of current episode; other mood or psychotic symptoms; current substance use **Past psychiatric History:** Prior episodes (number of episodes, duration, average severity, time since last episode); other psychiatric disorders; substance use; medication trials **Past Medical History:** Include seizures, symptoms of seizure, tremor, brain tumor/malignancy, neurological disorders; heat/cold intolerance, thyroid disorders; HIV or STIs **Medications:** Include current medications and compliance **Family History:** Include family history of bipolar disorder, MDD, schizophrenia, neurological disorders such as seizures, Huntington's, or multiple sclerosis **Social History:** Include risky behaviors such as unsafe sex or intravenous drug use **Review of Systems:** Include seizure symptoms; focal weakness, headaches, nausea (to assess for neurological illness); joint pain, photosensitivity, rash (to assess for SLE)
General Medical and Neurologic Examination with special attention to:
Look for signs of intoxication/withdrawal; thyroid abnormalities (sweating, tachycardia, atrial fibrillation, tremor); increased intracranial pressure (ocular abnormalities); strokes (focal weakness, sensory disturbances); SLE (malar rash, oral ulcers)
Psychiatric Mental Status Examination with special attention to:
Grooming (e.g. excessive makeup, revealing clothing); excitability; pressured speech; expansive, irritable, or labile mood/affect; disorganized thoughts (loosening of associations, flight of ideas); grandiose delusions; psychotic symptoms; impaired insight/judgment
Laboratory Studies, Imaging, and Other Diagnostic Tools with special attention to:
First-line: Toxicology screen, TSH, CBC, Chem7, UA Head CT recommended once for newly diagnosed patients (not needed acutely) **Second-line, if indicated:** HIV (if high-risk), RPR (if high-risk)

TABLE 3-18 Suggested Treatment by Mood Subtype

Dysphoric or mixed mania	Valproate or atypical antipsychotics; ECT
Severe mania or bipolar depression in pregnancy	ECT
Rapid-cycling (at least four mood episodes within 12 months)	Initially lithium or valproate; alternatively lamotrigine
Bipolar depression	Quetiapine, combination of olanzapine and fluoxetine (first choice, FDA approved; antidepressant monotherapy not recommended due to concerns for induced mania), ECT, lithium, or lamotrigine (for severe depression, may initiate lithium AND lamotrigine)

Obsessions and Compulsions

Freud believed that unacceptable emotions and ideas resulted in the development of obsessions and compulsions, leading to a patient's gradual withdrawal from society. Although these symptoms are often extremely disabling for patients, psychiatrists can effectively treat these patients effectively with different modalities of psychotherapy and psychopharmacology.

Definitions

- **Obsession:** recurrent, intrusive thought, feeling, or sensation
- **Compulsion:** conscious, standard, recurrent behavior or mental behavior (e.g., counting, checking, praying, avoiding) to alleviate distress in response to obsession. Compulsions do not always succeed in reducing anxiety

TABLE 3-19 Differential Diagnosis of Obsessions and Compulsions

Nonpsychiatric Conditions	
• Tourette's syndrome • Other tic disorders • Temporal lobe epilepsy	• Trauma • Postencephalitic complications
Psychiatric Conditions	
• OCD • Schizophrenia • Specific phobia • Obsessive-compulsive personality disorder	• Major depression • Hypochondriasis • Body dysmorphic disorder • Trichotillomania • Other impulse control disorders

OCD, obsessive–compulsive disorder

TABLE 3-20 Approach to the Evaluation of Obsessions and Compulsions

History with special attention to:

Common chief complaints:
- Can't leave the house
- Chapped hands
- Brought in by family for compulsions
- Concerns about "abnormal" physical features
- Anxiety
- Getting "stuck"

Symptom clusters:
- **Contamination:** fears of infection or germs followed by washing or avoidance of source of contamination
- **Pathological doubt:** obsession of doubt followed by a compulsion of checking to alleviate guilt or fear of danger
- **Intrusive thoughts:** intrusive obsessional thoughts without associated compulsion, often involving sex or violence
- **Symmetry:** need for symmetry or precision; leads to compulsion of being extremely slow because of ordering and arranging
- **Scrupulosity:** excessive praying or religious concerns exceeding the magnitude appropriate to patient's religious, family, or cultural context
- **Hoarding:** hoarding and collecting various objects more than is appropriate to the patient's context

Associated psychiatric symptoms: the most common comorbidities are depression (67%) and social phobia (25%)

Medical and surgical history: group A beta-hemolytic streptococcal infection may cause rheumatic fever; 10%–30% of patients develop Sydenham's chorea and OCD symptoms

Psychiatric history: previous behavioral and pharmacologic treatments

General Medical and Neurologic examination with special attention to:

Chapped hands, bald patches, skin picking (to assess for compulsive behaviors), vocal tics, motor tics, and chorea (to assess for tic disorders)

Psychiatric Mental Status Examination with special attention to:

Obsessions, overt compulsions, mental compulsions (checking, praying, or other mental rituals), intrusive thoughts with sexual or violent content, feelings of dread or urgency, avoidance behaviors, insight (may vary)

Laboratory Studies, Imaging, and Other Diagnostic Tools with special attention to:

First-line studies: EEG only if suspicious of a seizure disorder

Second-line studies, if indicated: CT and MRI have been used in research but are not indicated for clinical use

CT, computed tomography; EEG, electroencephalography; MRI, magnetic resonance imaging; OCD, obsessive–compulsive disorder.

Obsessive–Compulsive Disorder

- Characterized by symptoms of recurrent obsessions or compulsions that cause marked distress to the patient (time consuming; interfere with functioning)
- Both obsessions and compulsions are ego dystonic
- Intrusive thoughts, impulses, or images are not excessive worries about "real-life" problems; the patient realizes they are a product of his or her mind

Treatment

Therapy

- Behavior therapy is effective in significantly reducing symptoms. Examples include exposure-response prevention, flooding, desensitization, thought stopping, implosion therapy, and aversive conditioning
- Psychodynamic therapy may be helpful in understanding the meaning of the symptoms to the patient and may help when there is resistance to treatment
- Family, group, and couples therapy may also be helpful

Pharmacotherapy

- **SSRIs:** approved for treatment of OCD; higher dosages than usual are needed; best in combination with psychotherapy
  - Fluvoxamine: 50–300 mg
  - Paroxetine: 10–60 mg
  - Sertraline: 50–300 mg
  - Fluoxetine: 20–80 mg
- **Clomipramine:** most selective for serotonin reuptake; first drug approved for treatment of OCD; titrated up over 2–3 weeks; best combined with therapy
  - Dose: 25–250 mg
  - Watch for anticholinergic side effects and sedation
- **Other drugs** (less evidence of effectiveness)
  - Mood stabilizers: valproate, lithium, or carbamazepine
  - Atypical antipsychotics: olanzapine, risperidone, or quetiapine
  - Other antidepressants: venlafaxine, duloxetine, or MAOIs
  - Other medications: buspirone, benzodiazepines
- Rare treatments for treatment-resistant OCD: electroconvulsive therapy (ECT), psychosurgery (cingulotomy is most common)

EPIDEMIOLOGY/ETIOLOGY

- 2%–3% of the general population
- Same across cultural boundaries
- Men = women
- Mean age of onset: ~20 years
- Most support for serotonin dysregulation hypothesis
- Neuroimaging: altered function in circuits between orbitofrontal cortex, caudate, and thalamus
- Positron emission computed tomography: increased activity in the frontal lobes and basal ganglia
- Monozygotic > dizygotic twins

EXPOSURE-RESPONSE PREVENTION

- Most effective behavioral intervention
- Graded exposure to anxiety-provoking stimuli
- *Sample hierarchy for contamination:*
  - Limited number of handwashes
  - Sitting next to someone sick
  - Touching a toilet seat
  - Holding a biohazard box
  - Touching someone's blood

Personality Disorders

Every individual has a discrete pattern of behavior that characterizes his or her distinct personality. When personality types are considered pathologic, it is assumed that the pervasive and enduring patterns that comprise personality are maladaptive, and thus personality disorders represent "hopeless cases" that cannot be changed because of the inherent nature of one's personality. However, in recent years, with advances in research both validating effective treatments and elaborating the longitudinal course and neurobiologic, genetic, and environmental determinants of personality disorders, a new understanding of personality disorders as changeable, treatable, and in part biologically driven has emerged.

PERSONALITY DISORDERS (PD)

According to the *DSM-IV*, PDs are defined by patterns of behavior and enduring subjective experiences that deviate from cultural norms. They are pervasive and stable through time, leading to impairment and clinical distress. The *DSM-IV* also specifies that these patterns are manifest in two or more areas of cognition, affectivity, interpersonal functioning, and impulse control.

TABLE 3-21 Types of Personality Disorders

Personality Disorder (Prevalence)	Cognitive Features	Affective Features	Interpersonal Features	Behavioral Features
		Cluster A: "Weird" or "Eccentric"		
Paranoid (PPD) (0.5%–2.5%)	Reads hidden meanings into benign remarks or events		Mistrustful Suspicious Bears grudges	
Schizoid (SCD) (7.5%)		Emotionally cold Flat	Uninterested in others and relationships	
Schizotypal (SPD) (3%)	Ideas of reference Magical and odd thinking Body illusions Paranoid ideation	Inappropriate and constricted Socially anxious	Lacks close relationships other than first-degree relatives	Odd Eccentric
		Cluster B: "Wild" or "Dramatic"		
Antisocial (APD) (3% in men; 1% in women)		Lack of remorse Irritability	Failure to conform to social norms Deceitful Reckless	Impulsive Fails to plan ahead Irresponsible

(continued)

TABLE 3-21 Types of Personality Disorders (*continued*)

Personality Disorder (Prevalence)	Cognitive Features	Affective Features	Interpersonal Features	Behavioral Features
Cluster B: "Wild" or "Dramatic"				
Borderline (BPD) (1%–2%; ≤20% of psychiatric patients; more prevalent in females)	Transient, stress-related paranoia or dissociation	Affective instability Chronic emptiness Intense anger	Frantic efforts to avoid abandonment Unstable, intense relationships	Impulsive Recurrent suicidal behavior or self-mutilating behavior
Histrionic (HPD) (2%–3%)	Suggestible	Expression of emotion is rapidly shifting, shallow, and exaggerated	Seductive Provocative Attention seeking	Dramatic Theatrical
Narcissistic (NPD) (1%; 16% in psychiatric patients)	Grandiose sense of self-importance Preoccupied with fantasies of unlimited success	Envious Arrogant	Requires excessive admiration Entitled Exploitative Lacks empathy	
Cluster C: "Worried" or "Anxious"				
Avoidant (APD) (1%–10%)	Views self as inept, unappealing, and inferior		Socially inhibited Hypersensitive to negative evaluation	Avoids taking risks out of fear of embarrassment
Dependent (DPD)		Helpless and fearful when alone	Submissive Clinging Difficulty expressing disagreement	Difficulty initiating activity independent of others
Obsessive–compulsive (OCPD) (1%; 3%–10% of psychiatric patients)	Preoccupation with orderliness and perfection Scrupulous Inflexibility		Preoccupied with interpersonal control Excessive devotion to work at expense of friendships Reluctant to delegate tasks	Preoccupation with order and perfectionism interferes with task completion Unable to discard worn-out or worthless objects

PATHOPHYSIOLOGY

- **Biologic:**
  - The importance of genetic factors has been demonstrated through numerous family, twin, and adoption studies. Concordance for personality disorders is several times higher among monozygotic twins than dizygotic twins
  - Altered levels of neurotransmitters (serotonin, dopamine, endorphins, and other neuromodulatory agents) have been implicated in impulsivity, aggression, and other character traits
  - Other studies have identified platelet monoamine oxidase, smooth pursuit eye movements, and changes in electroencephalography (EEG) as possible correlates of personality disorders
- **Psychodynamic:**
  - Problems arise from conflicts and defenses based on Freud's topographic (conscious, preconscious, unconscious) or structural model (ego, superego, id). Symptoms based on maladaptive patterns of dealing with unconscious wishes and motives (*continued*)

TABLE 3-22 Approach to the Evaluation for Personality Disorders

History with special attention to:
History of present illness: onset (usually from young adulthood), symptoms, duration (ongoing and pervasive or temporary), other mood or psychotic symptoms, substance use, interpersonal stressors **Social history:** early attachments, living situation, important relationships, education, occupational functioning, religious and spiritual beliefs, trauma **Review of systems:** level of impairment and functioning
General **Medical** and **Neurologic examination** with special attention to:
Signs of eating disorder, self-injurious behavior, intoxication, or withdrawal
Psychiatric Mental Status Examination with special attention to:
Grooming, makeup, tattoos, piercings, clothing, level of engagement and eye contact, nervousness, labile mood or affect, fixed patterns or beliefs, thought patterns, odd behaviors, grandiosity, psychotic symptoms
Laboratory Studies, Imaging, and Other Diagnostic Tools with special attention to:
Obtain a head CT if there has been an abrupt change in pattern of behavior **Standardized assessments:** • **Clinician rated:** structured interview for *DSM-IV* Personality Disorders • Revised Diagnostic Interview for Borderlines • **Self-administered:** e.g., Minnesota Multiphasic Personality Inventory—Personality Disorder Scales, Millon Clinical Multiaxial Inventory—III

CT, computed tomography.

(*continued*)

- Ego psychology posits that patients with PD have deficits in functioning that limit their ability to use healthier defenses
- Self-psychology, object relations, attachment, and relational theories focus on an immature sense of self and internalization of inconsistent caretakers that lead to functional and relational difficulties

- **Cognitive-social:**
  - PD derived from learned behaviors and affective reactions associated with specific environmental contingencies

Treatment

- PDs improve at a significantly faster rate with psychotherapy compared with the natural course of illness
- Meta-analytic studies show both psychodynamic and CBT approaches are effective in the treatment of PDs
- **Borderline PD:** five empirically validated treatments that are all structured to stabilize the instability characteristic of BPD: dialectical behavior therapy (DBT), mentalization-based therapy (MBT), transference focused psychotherapy (TFP), schema-focused therapy (SFT), Systems Training for Emotional Predictability and Problem Solving (STEPPS)
- **Antisocial PD:** little efficacy with psychotherapy; some studies show worse outcomes

TABLE 3-23 Suggested Treatment of Personality Disorders

Treatment	Description
Psychotherapy	Psychodynamic, cognitive behavioral, individual, and group approaches. Focused on issues of managing affect and cognitions, self-image, and interpersonal relationships.
Pharmacotherapy	Treatment of comorbid Axis II disorders is necessary. In addition, anxiolytics, antipsychotics, antidepressants, mood stabilizers, and psychostimulants may be beneficial.

Problems with Sexual Function and Behaviors

Sexual symptoms may be challenging to identify because there is a broad range of what is considered "normal." Individual sexual experience is diverse, emerging from a combination of biologic factors, personal relational history, and community influence. The symptoms described here refer to patterns of sexual experience that may be associated with significant psychological distress. It is not intended to imply that the phenomena are inherently pathologic. For clinicians, an empathic approach to sexuality should focus on addressing patient distress and impaired function.

TABLE 3-24 Differential Diagnosis of Sexual Function and Behaviors

Nonpsychiatric Conditions
Medical and surgical conditions, side effects of illicit drugs or alcohol, and medications
Psychiatric Conditions
Paraphilias • **Sexual dysfunction disorders** • **Gender identity disorder** • **Other psychiatric disorders:** depression, bipolar manic episodes, anxiety disorders, OCD, schizophrenia, mental retardation, dementia, substance intoxication, personality disorder • **Psychological issues:** fears of intimacy or commitment, interpersonal conflict • **Nonparaphiliac compulsive sexual behaviors:** compulsive use of pornography via videos, magazines, or the Internet; uncontrolled masturbation, cybersex, unrestrained use of prostitutes • **Hypersexuality or sex addiction**

OCD, obsessive–compulsive disorder.

PARAPHILIA

- **Definition:** Recurrent, intense sexually arousing urges, fantasies, or behaviors that involve atypical objects, activities, or situations
  - The diagnosis is made only if associated with clinically significant distress or impairment in functioning, with symptoms lasting at least 6 months
  - Care must be taken to distinguish from nonpathologic use of sexual fantasies, behaviors, or objects used for sexual excitement
  - Significant distress or impairment may manifest as a behavior that is obligatory, causes sexual dysfunction, involves nonconsenting individuals, creates legal difficulties, or causes relationship difficulties

Treatment Considerations

- Patients rarely seek treatment voluntarily
  - They are usually mandated by a legal authority or persuaded by family to seek treatment
  - The paraphilia is a means to intense pleasure and is often extremely difficult to stop
- Specialized treatment is warranted and may include:
  - Psychological (e.g., behavioral therapies and CBT groups)
  - Biological approaches (e.g., testosterone-lowering medications)

TABLE 3-25 Approach to the Evaluation of Problems with Sexual Function and Behavior

History with special attention to:

Patients may be secretive because of shame, embarrassment, or legal ramifications. Use open-ended questions and avoid preconceived statements and opinions.

General
- Age, sex, occupation, sexual orientation
- Relationships (status, history, current and past dating activity)

Current Functioning
- Unsatisfactory? Why? Perception of partner satisfaction
- Specific dysfunctions
- Frequency of sexual activity (partnered or masturbation) and of sexual desire (feelings, thoughts, fantasy, dreams)
- Sense of compulsivity? Intrusion of sexual thoughts or activities interfering with relations, work, or safety or requiring deception?

Childhood Sexuality
- Parental attitudes, sources of sex education (e.g., structured, magazines, friends), first exposures to sexual situations

Adolescent and Adult Sexuality
- Age and reaction to pubertal onset (menarche or semenarche)
- Sense of self as masculine or feminine and desirable
- Patterns of masturbation (age of onset, frequency, fantasies, punishments or prohibition)
- Homosexual or heterosexual activities, experiences of dating, physical affection
- Orgasms (during masturbation, sleep, or with partner)
- First coitus (age, circumstances, experience, contraception, disease prevention)
- Types and number of partners

Special Issues
- Assume that sexual history continues to develop after widowhood, separation, and divorce
- History of rape, incest, physical or sexual abuse, current abuse
- Chronic illness (physical or psychiatric), STD, fertility, abortion or miscarriage, gender identity issues, paraphilias

General Medical and Neurologic examination with special attention to:

Endocrine, neurologic, and vascular function

Psychiatric Mental Status examination with special attention to:

Symptoms of concurrent conditions

Laboratory Studies, Imaging, and Other Diagnostic Tools with special attention to:

- Lipids, thyroid function, fasting blood sugar, endocrine (testosterone, prolactin, LH, FSH, estrogen, vaginal smear, MRI), ESR, Pap smear, nocturnal penile tumescence studies, ultrasonography, angiography
- Refer to medical subspecialties as necessary

ESR, erythrocyte sedimentation rate; FSH, follicle-stimulating hormone; LH, luteinizing hormone; MRI, magnetic resonance imaging; STD, sexually transmitted disease.

TABLE 3-26 Types of Paraphilias

Disorder	Sexual Arousal Related to:	Considerations
Exhibitionism	Exposing one's genitals to unsuspecting strangers	• May masturbate before, during, or after exposure • Reward is to shock the victim. • Unlikely to pursue the victim • Onset is typically before age 18 years
Fetishism	Use of nonliving objects, known as the "fetish," for fantasy, masturbation, or partnered encounters	• Most commonly women's undergarments, shoes, and apparel • Onset is typically during adolescence • Diagnosis is not made if accounted for by transvestic fetishism (cross-dressing) or if an object is used to stimulate the genitals (e.g., a vibrator)
Frotteurism	Touching and rubbing against a nonconsenting person	• Often occurs in crowded public places where the behavior can be engaged in surreptitiously
Pedophilia	Sexual activity with a prepubescent child (patient must be at least 16 years of age and 5 years older than the victim)	• Most commonly identified paraphilia • Most often heterosexual, with female targets or relatives
Sexual sadism	Sexual arousal derived from causing mental or physical suffering to a nonconsenting person	• More often seen in men • May be diagnosed if the patient presents with sexual sadistic fantasy • If the fantasy is acted on with nonconsenting person, the behavior is likely to be repeated
Sexual masochism	Sexual arousal derived from being the recipient of physical or mental abuse or humiliation	• In some cases, it is associated with dangerous practices such as autoerotic asphyxia (oxygen deprivation to enhance arousal)
Transvestic fetishism	Sexual arousal from cross-dressing in a heterosexual male	• The wife or female partner may be aware and may assist in selecting clothes or seeking treatment
Voyeurism	Watching an unsuspecting person who is naked, disrobing, or engaging in sexual activity	• Most commonly seen in men • Masturbation is commonly associated with voyeuristic behavior
Paraphilia NOS	Does not meet criteria for any of the above categories Examples: telephone scatologia (obscene phone calls), necrophilia (corpses), partialism (exclusive focus on a part of the body), zoophilia (animals), coprophilia (feces), klismaphilia (enemas), and urophilia (urine)	• There are more than 50 named paraphilias in the sexologic literature • Some of these paraphilias appear to be quite rare, but others seem relatively common • They includes the nondeviant sexual disorders such as compulsive masturbation and Internet pornography addiction

NOS, not otherwise specified.

SEXUAL DYSFUNCTION

- Definition: a disturbance in sexual desire and related psychophysiologic changes of the sexual response cycle (see Table 3-27) that causes marked distress and interpersonal difficulty
- DSM-IV categories:
  1. Sexual desire disorders (hypoactive or aversion)
  2. Sexual arousal disorders
  3. Orgasmic disorders (female; male premature ejaculation)
  4. Sexual pain disorders (dyspareunia, vaginismus)
  5. Sexual dysfunction caused by a general medical condition
  6. Substance-induced sexual dysfunction
  7. Sexual dysfunction NOS

SPECIFY IF THE CONDITION IS

- Lifelong (since onset of sexual functioning) or acquired
- Generalized or situational
- Caused by psychological or combined factors (psychological and caused by a general medical condition or substance induced)

TABLE 3-27 Sexual Response Cycle and Related Sexual Dysfunctions

Stage	Definition	Related Dysfunction
1. Desire	Fantasies and desire to have sexual activity	• Hypoactive sexual desire disorder • Sexual aversion disorder
2. Excitement	Subjective sexual pleasure and physiologic changes (penile tumescence and erection, vaginal lubrication and expansion and vasocongestion of the external genitalia)	• Female sexual arousal disorder • Male erectile disorder • Dyspareunia caused by a general medical condition
3. Orgasm	Peaking sexual pleasure, release of sexual tension, and rhythmic contraction of the perineal muscles and reproductive organs; ejaculation of semen in males	• Female orgasmic disorder • Male orgasmic disorder • Premature ejaculation • General medical condition • Substance-induced sexual dysfunction with impaired orgasm
4. Resolution	Muscular relaxation, sense of general well-being; in males, a refractory period to further erection and orgasm	• Postcoital dysphoria • Postcoital headache

Treatment Considerations

- **Psychological and behavioral treatment**
  - Reassurance
  - Education

- Technical suggestions
  - "Sensate focus" exercises (focus on sense experience rather than on a goal of orgasm)
  - Exploration with fantasy
  - Physical maneuvers (e.g., Kegel exercises, manual stimulation for female orgasmic disorder, or the "squeeze technique" for premature ejaculation)
- **Organic treatments**
  - Treat pre-existing illnesses (e.g., diabetes), screen for medications or illicit drugs that are associated with sexual side effects, and correct hormone deficiencies
  - For **premature ejaculation,** consider prescribing medications that have been associated with delayed ejaculation (e.g., fluoxetine)
  - For **erectile dysfunction,** consider phosphodiesterase-5 inhibitors (sildenafil, vardenafil, tadalafil; note contraindication with nitrates)
  - Additional organic treatments likely involve consultation with a specialist

GENDER IDENTITY DISORDERS

- **Definition:** Strong and persistent cross-gender identification (not merely an opportunistic desire for perceived cultural advantages of the other gender) that is accompanied by lasting discomfort with one's assigned gender or sense of appropriateness in the gender role of that gender. The disorder often begins in childhood and has a chronic course that may develop into transsexualism
- **Terminology**
  - **Gender identity:** self-perception as a male or female
  - **Gender dysphoria:** discomfort with one's assigned gender and desire to have the body of the other gender and be regarded by others as a member of the other gender
  - Sex = anatomical and physiological gender
  - Sexual orientation = erotic attraction to males, females, or both
  - Transsexual = persistent preoccupation with removing or acquiring secondary sex characteristics of the other gender
- **Differential diagnosis**
  - Transvestic fetishism: cross-dressing for sexual excitement
  - Psychotic disorders: delusion
  - Intersexual disorders: biologically based syndromes such as Turner's syndrome, Klinefelter's syndrome, androgen insensitivity syndrome, hermaphroditism
- **Treatment**
  - Psychotherapy to become comfortable with the desired gender identity
  - Consideration of a trial of cross-dressing
  - Exploration of hormone replacement therapy, sex reassignment surgery, or both

Psychosis

Psychosis is a symptom of severe psychiatric and nonpsychiatric disorders that may be short lived or chronic. Often misunderstood, affected individuals face a debilitating break in reality that influences all aspects of their lives. Whatever the cause, psychosis requires prompt evaluation and treatment, often including hospitalization and pharmacologic treatments.

DEFINITION

- A **break from reality,** as evidenced by delusions, hallucinations, illusions, disordered thinking, loss of ego boundaries, or failed reality testing
- Affects **thought content** (paranoid delusions, ideas of reference) or **thought process** (tangentiality, loose associations, thought blocking)
- A **symptom** of various disorders but not a disorder itself
- Lifetime prevalence of 3% in the United States (Perala et al, 2007)

TABLE 3-28 Differential Diagnosis of Psychosis

Nonpsychiatric Conditions
Prescription Medications • Anticholinergic agents, digitalis toxicity, glucocorticoids, ACTH, isoniazid, L-Dopa and other dopamine agents, NSAIDs, MAOI withdrawal **Illicit Drugs** • Withdrawal: alcohol, sedative-hypnotics • Intoxication: amphetamines, cocaine, PCP, ketamine, hallucinogens **Medical Conditions** • Complex partial seizures (auras, automatisms), CNS infection, neurosyphilis, brain tumor, SLE (tactile and visual hallucinations), Huntington's disease, Wilson's disease • Metabolic abnormalities, thyroid disease, parathyroid disease, nutritional deficiencies, toxins

Psychiatric Conditions	
• Schizophrenia	• Culture-specific psychoses
• Schizophreniform	• Mental retardation
• Schizoaffective disorder	• OCD
• Brief psychotic disorder	• Autistic disorder
• Shared psychotic disorder (Folie a deux)	• Malingering • Factitious disorder
• Delusional disorder	• Personality disorders, particularly schizotypal, schizoid, borderline, paranoid
• Bipolar disorder with psychotic features	
• Major depression with psychotic features	• Narcolepsy (daytime hypnagogic or -pompic hallucinations)

ACTH, adrenocorticotropic hormone; CNS, central nervous system; MAOI, monoamine oxidase inhibitor; NSAID, nonsteroidal antiinflammatory drug; OCD, obsessive–compulsive disorder; PCP, phencyclidine; SLE, systemic lupus erythematosus.

TABLE 3-29 Approach to the Evaluation for Psychosis

History with special attention to:

Source: obtain collateral information from family, friends, and treaters
Social history: include birth history and developmental history
Review of systems: include environmental exposures and nutritional deficiencies

General Medical and Neurologic Examination with special attention to:

Motor abnormalities (TD, Parkinsonism, akathisia, NMS)

Psychiatric Mental Status with special attention to:

Level of functioning declines or is below expected level
Abnormal though content:

- **Delusions:** fixed, false beliefs based on an incorrect inference about an external reality that fail to correct with reasoning and are inconsistent with the patient's culture and education
- **Ideas of reference:** words or actions that have personal, special meaning but not full delusional properties (e.g., license plate of passing car is evidence of a conspiracy against the person)

Distorted perception:

- **Hallucinations:** sensory experiences in the absence of an inciting stimulus that are not under the person's control
- **Illusions:** misinterpretation of existing sensory stimulus

Illogical thought processes: Circumstantiality, tangentiality, derailment, loose associations, word salad, clang association, thought blocking, echolalia, neologisms
Affect: flat, blunted, labile, inappropriate
Impaired sense of self: loss of ego boundaries, inability to distinguish internal and external reality
Psychomotor behavior: abnormal, agitation, aggression, violence risk, withdrawal, catatonia, posturing
Cognition: impaired: concrete, inattentive, poor information processing

Laboratory Studies, Imaging, and Other Diagnostic Tools with special attention to:

First-line studies: CBC, electrolytes, BUN or creatinine, glucose, calcium, phosphate, TSH, LFTs, HIV screen, FTA-Abs (RPR not sufficient), vitamin B12, folate, UA, urine drug screen, MRI (to rule out masses, demyelinating disease, mesial temporal lobe sclerosis)
Second-line studies, if indicated: ESR, ANA, ceruloplasmin, EEG, genetic tests, lumbar puncture, neuropsychological testing

ANA, antinuclear antibody; BUN, blood urea nitrogen; CBC, complete blood count; EEG, electroencephalography; ESR, erythrocyte sedimentation rate; FTA-Abs, fluorescent treponema antibody test; HIV, human immunodeficiency virus; LFT, liver function test; MRI, magnetic resonance imaging; NMS, neuroleptic malignant syndrome; RPR, rapid plasma regain; TD, tardive dyskinesia; TSH, thyroid-stimulating hormone; UA, urinalysis.

SCHIZOPHRENIA (SCZ)

- Seen in **functionally impaired** patients with at least **two characteristic symptoms** (delusions, hallucinations, disorganized speech, disorganized or catatonic behavior, or negative symptoms) with effects lasting at least **6 months**
- Symptoms understood categorically (*DSM-IV-TR*):
  - **Positive:** an excess or distortion of normal functions; involves a "psychotic dimension" (delusions, hallucinations) or a "disorganization dimension" (disorganized speech and behavior, catatonia)
  - **Negative:** a diminution or loss of normal functions; involves decreased emotional expressivity (affective flattening), restricted speech fluency or thought production (alogia), and reduced goal-directed behavior (a volition)
- Most common: delusions (persecutory and referential) and hallucinations (auditory)
- Disorganized thinking (formal thought disorder) that impairs effective communication
- Disorganized behavior without understandable motivations
- Catatonic behavior: motoric immobility, excessive motor activity, extreme negativism, mutism, peculiarities of voluntary movement, echolalia, or echopraxia

EPIDEMIOLOGY
- Prevalence: ~1% worldwide; male > female
- Onset: men: 18–25 years old; women: 25 years to mid 30s; late-onset 45 years; very late onset >60 years
- Urban born > rural born

TABLE 3-26 Schizophrenia Subtypes

Subtype	Characteristics
Paranoid	Delusions or auditory hallucinations No prominent negative symptoms or disorganization
Disorganized	Disorganized speech and behavior with flat or inappropriate affect but does not meet criteria for catatonic type
Catatonic	Must have two symptoms, including waxy flexibility or stupor, excessive motor activity, extreme negativism or mutism, peculiar voluntary movements, echolalia, or echopraxia
Undifferentiated	Has positive symptoms but does not the meet criteria for above
Residual	No positive symptoms but continued evidence of negative symptoms

Treatment

- Antipsychotic choice for maintenance treatment
  - Clozapine has the greatest efficacy but a severe side effect profile; it is used for refractory patients
  - Efficacy studies show no clear differences between second-generation (atypical) antipsychotics (Motlová a et al, 2007)

- Psychosocial interventions
  - Early intervention programs improve outcome
  - Consider psychoeducation, social skills training, family therapy, group therapy, individual psychotherapy (supportive, CBT, psychodynamic), vocational rehabilitation, and self-help groups
  - Patients may benefit from structured living situations or long-term inpatient care

Schizophreniform

- Meets criteria for SCZ but lasts only **1 to 6 months**
- Impaired social or occupational functioning is not necessary for diagnosis
- Approximately one third of individuals recover in 6 months and two thirds progress to SCZ or schizoaffective disorder
- Good prognostic indicators: psychotic symptom onset within 1 month of the first behavioral changes, confusion at the peak of the psychotic episode, good premorbid functioning, lack of flat affect
- Treatment is similar to treatment for SCZ

Schizoaffective Disorder

- Meets criteria for SCZ along with major depressive, manic, or mixed episodes
  - Delusions or hallucinations must occur for at least **2 weeks without prominent mood symptoms**
  - Mood symptoms must be present for a significant portion of the illness
- Prognosis is better than for SCZ but worse than for mood disorders
- Treatment includes antipsychotics with or without concurrent antidepressants or mood stabilizers for mood symptoms

Brief Psychotic Disorder

- Abrupt onset (usually the late 20s or early 30s) of at least **one positive psychotic symptom** lasting **1 day to 1 month** often in response to stress with return to premorbid functioning with treatment or removal of the stressor
- Responsive to antipsychotics

Shared Psychotic Disorder (Folie a Deux)

- Occurs when delusion develops in a person involved in a close relationship with another person ("the inducer" or "the primary case") who already has a delusion, and the two are relatively isolated from other social contacts
- Treatment often requires antipsychotics and separation of the enmeshed pair

Delusional Disorder

- Typically **high-functioning** patients with isolated, **nonbizarre delusions** (culturally defined, plausible) that **are well systematized** (all logically fit a complex scheme) lasting at least **1 month**

- Onset is insidious and typically occurs in midlife; lifetime prevalence is estimated at 0.03%
- Hallucinations are not prominent but olfactory or tactile hallucinations consistent with the delusion (e.g., smelling poison being pumped into room, parasites crawling on skin) may be seen
- Treatment includes antipsychotic medications, but response is less robust than with other psychotic disorders

TREATMENT OF PSYCHOSIS

- Acute issues:
  - **Antipsychotic medication** is warranted to prevent injury to oneself or others
  - **Inpatient hospitalization** should be considered for initial assessment, initiation of treatment, risk of harm to oneself or others, inability to care for oneself, treatment of severe antipsychotic side effects, and ECT
- General antipsychotic considerations:
  - Overall goal: **control of symptoms** on **monotherapy** with the **lowest effective dose**
  - Effective trial time is **2 to 3 months** at **therapeutic dosing** range; full effect may take 6 months
  - Goal dosing: ranges must be flexible; there is no clear relationship between dose and effectiveness
- Antipsychotic choice in general:
  - Efficacy studies show no proven differences except for clozapine
  - Consider side effects, prior response, medical comorbidities, drug interactions, tolerability, patient preference, and dosing forms available (e.g., intramuscular [IM], dissolving tablets)
  - First-generation (typical) antipsychotics or second-generation (atypical) antipsychotics are indicated
  - For **rapid onset,** consider an IM formulation (chlorpromazine, haloperidol, fluphenazine, perphenazine, olanzapine, ziprasidone, aripiprazole) or an IV formulation (haloperidol)
  - For **adherence** as a primary issue, try a **long-acting formulation** (haloperidol, fluphenazine, risperidone)
  - For **failure of more than two antipsychotics** with effective trials, clozapine is effective in 30% to 60% of nonresponders (Kane, 1992). Clozapine is superior to other antipsychotic agents in efficacy but is not a first-line choice because of serious side effects
  - Consider ECT in refractory patients and those with severe mood symptoms
  - Monitor for neuroleptic malignant syndrome, acute dystonia (may be fatal), and dose-related EPS
  - Assess for QTc prolongation (risk of torsades) when indicated
  - Use of antipsychotics in pregnant patients is unclear. There is possible teratogenicity, risk of neonatal EPS, or effects in breast milk. The best evidence of safety is for first-generation (typical) antipsychotics

- Other medications to consider:
  - Adjunctive as-needed benzodiazepines for the first week may help agitation
  - Divalproex or carbamazepine may help with agitation, aggressiveness, and manic-like symptoms (note: carbamazepine lowers clozapine levels)
  - Antidepressants may help depressive symptoms
  - Consider prophylactic dystonia treatment (highest risk in young Asian American males with a history of EPS)
    - Benztropine: 2 mg PO twice a day (BID) or 1 mg PO BID if anticholinergic side effects are present.

Sleep Disorders

The following is not a comprehensive list of all sleep disorders, but rather a brief primer on common sleep disorders seen in psychiatric practice. If one of the following primary sleep disorders is suspected, referral to a sleep medicine specialist for further workup and management is frequently warranted, particularly if polysomnography (PSG) is indicated.

TABLE 3-31 Differential Diagnosis of Sleep Disorders

Disorders of Initiation and Maintenance of Sleep
- Insomnia
- RLS
- Circadian rhythm sleep disorders

Disorders of Excessive Daytime Sleepiness
- Voluntary sleep deprivation
- SRBDs
- Narcolepsy

Parasomnias
- NREM parasomnias
- REM parasomnias

NREM, non–rapid eye movement; REM, rapid eye movement; RLS, restless legs syndrome; SRBD, sleep-related breathing disorder.

Disorders of Initiation and Maintenance of Sleep

Insomnia

DEFINITION

Symptoms of difficulty initiating or maintaining sleep, early awakenings, or nonrestorative sleep despite adequate opportunities for sleep

- **Insomnia disorder:** insomnia symptoms with significant distress or impairment
- **Primary insomnia:** insomnia with no clear medical or psychiatric cause

(*continued*)

TABLE 3-32 Approach to the Evaluation of Sleep Complaints

History with special attention to:

Chief complaint: primary sleep complaint (e.g., excessive daytime sleepiness, insomnia, parasomnia)

History of present illness: a detailed sleep history covers a patient's signs and symptoms over a 24-hour day

- Pattern, onset, history, course, duration, severity of sleep complaint
- Factors that exacerbate or improve symptoms:, response to prior treatment, self-help attempts
- Daytime sleepiness should be differentiated from fatigue with careful questioning
- Bedtime factors: routines, behaviors, bodily sensations, cognitive arousal, sleep latency
- Nighttime factors: snoring, witnessed apneas, nocturnal awakenings, parasomnias
- Daytime factors: wake time, daytime sleepiness, hyperarousal, cataplexy, naps, exercise, caffeine use, daily activities
- Changes in daily or nightly routines: weekend variation

Medical history: medical disorders associated with sleep disruption (e.g., Parkinson's disease, CHF, prostatic hypertrophy, pain syndromes)

Family history: focus on primary sleep disorders, including RLS, sleep-disordered breathing, and narcolepsy as well as symptoms (e.g., EDS, snoring, insomnia) because family members also often have undiagnosed sleep disorders

Social history

- Presence or absence of a bed partner; if there is a bed partner, collateral information should be obtained
- Occupational, family, or social stressors that contribute to the sleep complaint

Review of systems: regardless of the sleep complaint, all patients should be screened for signs and symptoms of other primary sleep disorders

General Medical and Neurologic Examination with special attention to:

- Nasopharynx and oropharynx: degree of patency, adenotonsillar hypertrophy
- Retrognathia and micrognathia, dental malocclusion
- Neck circumference
- Evidence of parkinsonism if RBD is suspected

Psychiatric Mental Status Examination with special attention to:

Presence of sleepiness during interview, limb movements, differentiation of daytime hallucinations from hypnogogic or -pompic

Laboratory Studies, Imaging, and Other Diagnostic Tests

- Referral to a sleep medicine specialist for further evaluation is often indicated
- Not all sleep disorders routinely require PSG for evaluation (e.g., insomnia, RLS, CRSD)
- PSG is indicated for suspected SRBD
- PSG with MSLT (nap study that objectively assesses daytime sleepiness) is indicated for workup of suspected CNS hypersomnias (e.g., narcolepsy)
- Patients with suspected RLS should be evaluated with serum ferritin

CHF, congestive heart failure; CNS, central nervous system; CRSD, circadian rhythm sleep disorder; EDS, excessive daytime sleepiness; MSLT, multiple sleep latency test; PSG, polysomnography; RBD, rapid eye movement behavior disorder; RLS, restless legs syndrome; SRBD, sleep-related breathing disorder.

EPIDEMIOLOGY

- Most common sleep complaint in the general population
- 1-year prevalence of insomnia symptoms: 30%–40%; chronic insomnia: 5%–10% of the population

TREATMENTS

- Treat the underlying cause (e.g., medical or psychiatric illness) if present
- Treating insomnia and comorbid psychiatric illness may improve both
- **CBT for insomnia:**
  - Stimulus control: reassociate the sleeping environment with sleep (go to bed only when sleepy, leave bed if unable to sleep, use the bedroom for sleep only, do not take naps, keep a regular sleep–wake schedule)
  - Sleep restriction: time in bed is limited to the total number of hours slept and then gradually increased
  - Relaxation training: reduce somatic tension or intrusive thoughts at bedtime (e.g., muscle relaxation, meditation)
  - Cognitive therapy: challenge and change misconceptions about sleep and insomnia
  - Sleep hygiene education: guidelines regarding general health practices and environmental factors that may interfere with sleep
- **Pharmacotherapy** (see drug index for details)
  - Consider the half-life of the drug when selecting an agent; ideally, the drug would be present during sleep but eliminated by the time of wakefulness to minimize carry-over effects
  - Caution should be used in elderly individuals because of their decreased metabolism and increased adipose tissue may increase half-life
  - Other side effects (e.g., anticholinergic) on comorbid psychiatric illness should also be considered
  - Periodic discontinuation trials of sedative–hypnotics should be done in all patients when clinically feasible (Buysse et al, 2005)

Restless Legs Syndrome (RLS)

- **Definition:** sensorimotor disorder that presents because of sleep disruption with or without daytime sleepiness
- **Symptoms:** four essential diagnostic criteria (mnemonic "URGE"):
  - **U:** urge to move the limbs (with or without paresthesias)
  - **R:** rest induced
  - **G:** gets better with activity
  - **E:** evening and night accentuation

PATHOPHYSIOLOGY

- **Idiopathic:** dopaminergic dysfunction in subcortical systems and diminished central nervous system (CNS) iron
- **Secondary:** medical disorders (e.g., uremia, anemia) or medication induced (e.g., antidepressants, antipsychotics)
- **Related disorders:** periodic limb movements of sleep (PLMS) are often seen on PSG but are not pathognomic for RLS
- **Evaluation:** if serum ferritin is below 50 μg/L, testing should be repeated

(*continued*)

TABLE 3-33 Potential Pharmacologic Treatments for Insomnia*

Class of Drug	Name	Dosing Guidelines
BZRAs		
Selective for ∝-1 subunit on $GABA_A$ receptor	Zolpidem Zaleplon Eszopiclone	5–10 mg QHS 5–20 mg QHS 1–3 mg QHS
Nonselective benzodiazepines	Triazolam Lorazepam Temazepam	0.125–0.25 mg QHS 0.5–2.0 mg QHS 7.5–30 mg QHS
Sedating Antidepressants		
SSRI	Trazodone	12.5–100 mg QHS
TCAs	Doxepin Amitriptyline	10–50 mg QHS 10–50 mg QHS
Other	Mirtazapine	15–45 mg QHS
Antihistamines	Diphenhydramine	25–50 mg QHS
Antipsychotics	Quetiapine Olanzapine	12.5–100 mg QHS 2.5–5.0 mg QHS
Antiepileptic Drugs	Gabapentin Tiagabine	100–900 mg QHS 2–8 mg QHS
Melatonin Receptor Agonists	Ramelteon	8 mg PO QHS

*Only BZRAs and ramelteon have been approved by the Food and Drug Administration for the treatment of patients with primary insomnia; use of other agents is largely guided by clinical experience.

BZRA, benzodiazepine receptor agonist; GABA, γ-aminobutyric acid; QHS, at bedtime; SSRI, selective serotonin reuptake inhibitor; TCA, tricyclic antidepressant.

(*continued*)

TREATMENTS

- **Behavioral:** limit sleep deprivation, avoidance of caffeine and alcohol, and periods of immobility when possible
- **Pharmacologic:** dopamine agonists: (first line); ropinirole (0.25–4.00 mg) or pramipexole (0.125–0.75 mg) 2 hours before symptom onset; alternatives include gabapentin or opiates

Circadian Rhythm Sleep Disorders (CRSD)

Definition: disorders of the alteration of the phase relationship between intrinsic circadian system and extrinsic light–dark cycle, resulting in an abnormal and troublesome sleep–wake pattern

- Delayed sleep phase syndrome: bedtime and wake time (B + W) shifted late (e.g., 3 AM to 11 AM)
- Advanced sleep phase syndrome: B + W shifted early (e.g., 6 PM to 2 AM)
- Non–24-hour sleep–wake syndrome: B + W follows a non–24-hour (e.g., 25-hr) rhythm
- Irregular sleep–wake syndrome: lack of distinct sleep–wake cycles

- Shift work sleep disorder: insomnia or EDS caused by an enforced schedule (e.g., night shifts)
- Jet lag disorder: insomnia or EDS caused by time-zone shifts

Evaluation: clinical history with or without actigraphy (activity monitor worn on the wrist)

TREATMENT

Varies by disorder; light with or without melatonin at appropriate times, regular sleep–wake times

Disorders of Excessive Daytime Sleepiness

Voluntary Sleep Deprivation

- Most common cause of excessive daytime sleepiness

Sleep-Related Breathing Disorders (SRBDs)

- **Definition:** cessation of breathing (apnea) during sleep resulting in intermittent hypoxemia, arousals from sleep, or both
- **Symptoms:** EDS, snoring, witnessed apneas, fatigue, hypertension, diminished concentration, morning headaches, morning dry mouth, insomnia (occasionally), depression, irritability
- **Pathophysiology:** obstructive sleep apnea (OSA) caused by mechanical obstruction at the level of the upper airway; central sleep apnea (CSA) caused by a decreased CNS drive to breathe
- **Risk factors:** OSA (obesity, male, large neck circumference, crowded oropharynx, micrognathia, retrognathia); CSA (elderly, congestive heart failure, stroke, Cheyne-Stokes breathing, high altitudes, opiate use, acromegaly, hypothyroidism, and renal failure)
- **Evaluation:** PSG

Treatments

- **OSA:** Conservative measures (weight loss, avoidance of alcohol, maintaining nasal patency, avoidance of supine position during sleep); positive airway pressure (PAP) therapy (gold standard); oral appliance or upper airway surgery are alternatives
- **CSA:** Treatment of underlying cause of ventilatory instability (first line); PAP therapy, supplemental O_2, pharmacotherapy (e.g., acetazolamide or theophylline) may also be used

Narcolepsy

- **Definition:** CNS disorder affecting the sleep–wake cycle with EDS and symptoms of rapid eye movement (REM) sleep intrusion into wakefulness
- **Symptoms:** EDS, cataplexy (loss of muscle tone, particularly in response to emotional stimuli), hypnagogic or -pompic hallucinations, sleep paralysis, automatic behaviors
- **Pathophysiology:** loss of Orexin or hypocretin neurons in the lateral hypothalamus
- **Evaluation:** PSG and multiple sleep latency test (two or more sleep-onset REM periods are highly suggestive of diagnosis); additional tests may include HLA DQB1*0602 and cerebrospinal fluid Orexin; these are not routinely indicated

Treatments

- **Behavioral:** limit sleep deprivation; scheduled naps
- **Pharmacologic** (and target symptoms): stimulants (EDS), antidepressants (cataplexy), sodium oxybate (EDS with cataplexy)

Note: Other CNS hypersomnias (e.g., idiopathic hypersomnia) are beyond the scope of this manual. Please see Young and Silber (2006) for further details.

Parasomnias

- **Definition:** Disorders of undesirable physical or experiential events that occur during sleep; categorized by the stage of sleep from which the behavior or experience originates

NON–RAPID EYE MOVEMENT (NREM) PARASOMNIAS

In general, these parasomnias typically occur in the first 1 to 2 hours of the sleep period and are triggered by brief arousals to higher amplitude EEG ("disorders of arousal"). They occur along a spectrum of behavioral and affective expression; amnesia for the episode is typical.

- **Confusional arousals:** brief, simple motor behaviors occurring with minimal affective expression or responsiveness to the environment
- **Sleepwalking (somnambulism):** more complex motor behavior; can become violent if awakened suddenly; and common (≤20%) in children. They typically diminish by adulthood
- **Sleep terrors:** similar to sleepwalking but characterized by greater autonomic activity and affective expression. Common in children (5%) and characterized by a piercing scream followed by fear, crying, and inconsolability. They typically dissipate by adulthood
- **Other:** sleep-related eating disorder, sleep-related sexual behavior, and sleep-related violence

RAPID EYE MOVEMENT (REM) PARASOMNIAS

In general, these parasomnias are an inappropriate admixture of REM-related phenomena (atonia of skeletal muscles, dreaming, increased autonomic activity) and wakefulness.

- **REM behavior disorder (RBD):** failure of paralysis of skeletal muscles during REM sleep allows dream enactment; associated with synucleinopathies (e.g., Parkinson's disease)
- **Nightmare disorder:** recurrent dreams with emotions (fear, anger, embarrassment) and increased autonomic activity followed by awakening with full and often detailed recall of the dream; often leads to insomnia
- **Recurrent isolated sleep paralysis:** wakefulness at the onset or offset of sleep accompanied by paralysis of skeletal muscles with or without hypnopompic or -gogic hallucinations

Substance Use Disorders

Substance use disorders are among the most prevalent psychiatric disorders, affecting close to 10% of the US population. Identification and treatment of substance use disorders as well as frequently associated conditions, including psychiatric and medical illnesses, are crucial for the complete care of all patients.

Definitions and Diagnostic Criteria

Substance Abuse

Substance use causing significant impairment as manifested by at least one of the following over a 12-month period (and not meeting criteria for dependence):
- Neglect of responsibilities
- Legal problems
- Conflict with loved ones
- Jeopardizing personal health or safety

EPIDEMIOLOGY

General statistics (from the 2006 National Survey on Drug Use and Health)
- 9.2% of the US population has a substance use disorder
- 7.6% have an alcohol use disorder

Substance Dependence

Substance use causing significant impairment as manifested by at least three of the following over a 12-month period:
- Using more than intended
- Unsuccessful attempts to cut down or stop
- Neglect of responsibilities
- Spending a lot of time obtaining or using the substance
- Continued use despite awareness of harm to health or mental health
- Tolerance (need to use more to feel the same effect) or withdrawal symptoms: the presence of tolerance or withdrawal indicates physiologic dependence

Polysubstance Dependence

Use of at least three groups of substances in a pattern that meets criteria for substance dependence only when use of all substance types are considered together but not when each is considered individually
- A patient who fulfills dependence criteria for multiple individual substances independently has two or more different dependence disorders (e.g., alcohol dependence and opiate dependence)
- There is no such diagnosis as polysubstance abuse; a patient who abuses more than one substance has multiple different abuse disorders (only one criterion is necessary)

Treatment

Motivational Interviewing

"Preparing for Change"
- Therapeutic strategy to help patients who are less ready for change to enhance their intrinsic motivation to change. This is ideal for patients in the precontemplative or contemplative stages
- This is achieved by exploring and resolving the patient's own ambivalence
- Two phases:
  - Increasing the motivation to change
  - Solidifying the commitment to change
- Commitment strength during the final stages of therapy most strongly predicts behavior change. (The patient's starting level of motivation is not predictive.)
- Used as a brief, stand-alone intervention or combined with other treatment methods

TABLE 3-34 Approach to the Evaluation of Substance Abuse and Dependence

History with special attention to:

Substance use history: identify substances used and pattern of use
- Active screening for substance classes that are frequently underreported: steroids, prescription medications, cannabis
- Date of first use and last use
- Frequency, amount, and method of use (note: patients often underestimate)
- Other substances concurrently or previously used
- Dangerous substance combinations: use of an opioid plus a sedative–hypnotic may lead to respiratory depression; use of alcohol plus cocaine (cocaethylene metabolite) may lead to cardiotoxicity or an increased risk of stroke
- Review all criteria to determine abuse vs. dependence and harmful consequences attributable to substance use
- Assess the degree of physiologic dependence with the history of withdrawal symptoms (type, frequency, severity) and tolerance (increasing amount needed for intoxication, diminishment of pleasurable effects)

Treatment history: assess past treatments and interventions
- When and how many? (detoxification, residential or partial hospital, intensive outpatient, medications, AA/NA or other self-help, therapy, sober housing, needle exchange, drug court)
- Longest period sober
- Motivation to stay sober (past and present)
- Factors contributing to success and failure in the past

Psychiatric history: all psychiatric symptoms that pose a danger to the patient or a threat to achieving abstinence should be actively treated
- **Co-occurring psychiatric disorders:** symptoms predate substance use or persist during extended abstinence from substances
- **Substance-induced psychiatric disorders:** symptoms occur only in the context of use and exceed the expected psychoactive effects of intoxication or withdrawal; may persist in abstinence but generally diminish over time
- Screen for mood disorders, anxiety, PTSD, suicidality, self-injurious behavior, history of being intoxicated during SI or suicide attempts
- Screen for past psychiatric hospitalizations, past dual diagnosis hospitalizations

Medical History
- Actively screen for medical illnesses commonly co-occurring with substance use disorders: HCV, HBV, HIV, TB, MRSA, emphysema, pneumonia, cardiovascular events, sinusitis, hepatitis, gastritis, pancreatitis, injury-related trauma, neuropathies, seizures
- Injury sustained while operating motor craft or machinery under the influence of substances
- Hospitalizations for substance-related illnesses
- Victim or perpetrator of injuries because of violence while under the influence of substances

Family history
- Family members with history of substance use, relationship to patient (there is evidence of heritable vulnerability to both general and specific substance use disorders)
- Extent of use, abuse, and dependence by family members (predisposition to dependence is most strongly heritable)
- Treatment outcomes and complications of family members' use

(continued)

TABLE 3-34 Approach to the Evaluation of Substance Abuse and Dependence (*continued*)

Social history
- Housing, education, financial support, relationships, insurance status
- Significant figures in the patient's life and their involvement in his or her use; do they know of patient's drug use, encourage quitting, use themselves?
- Dependents: how have they been affected? Concern adequate to trigger filing with state social services?
- Relations with employer and coworkers
- Participation in self-help groups? Does the individual have an AA or NA sponsor?

Review of systems
Fevers, chills, weight and appetite, fatigue, abdominal pain or other GI symptoms, shortness of breath, cough, sexual dysfunction, sleep patterns, orthostasis, dizziness or ataxia, syncope, trauma, changes in distal sensation

General Medical and Neurologic Examination with special attention to:

- General: nutritional status, hygiene, odor, signs of fatigue
- Vital signs: tachycardia, high or labile blood pressure, oxygen saturation
- HEENT: nasal irritation or septum perforation, conjunctival injection or irritation, breath odor, stained teeth or dental erosion, perioral rash, thrush, cervical lymphadenopathy, pupillary size
- Cardiovascular: arrhythmias
- Lungs: findings of COPD
- Abdomen: tenderness, hepatomegaly
- Genital: warts, discharge, trauma, pap smear
- Extremities: signs of trauma, needle tracks, cellulitis, abscess
- Neurologic: neuropathies, nystagmus, ataxia, tremor

Psychiatric Mental Status Examination with special attention to:

Signs and symptoms of intoxication, withdrawal, stigma of chronic use

Laboratory Studies, Imaging, and Other Diagnostic Tests

First-line studies: toxicology screens (blood and urine), TSH, CBC, chemistry panel, UA, LFTs

Second-line studies, if indicated: pancreatic enzymes, HBV and HCV serologies, HIV test, MCV, GGT, CDT, PPD, CXR, PFTs, EKG, EEG, head CT or brain MRI

AA, alcoholics; CBC, complete blood count; CDT, carbohydrate-deficient transferring; Chem7 anonymous; COPD, chronic obstructive pulmonary disease; CT, computed tomography; CXR, chest radiography; EEG, electroencephalography; EKG, electrocardiography; GI, gastrointestinal; GGT, γ-glutamyl transferase; HBV, hepatitis B virus; HCV, hepatitis C virus; HEENT, head, eyes, ears, nose, and throat; HIV, human immunodeficiency virus; LFT, liver function test; MCV, mean corpuscular volume; MRI, magnetic resonance imaging; MRSA, methicillin-resistant *Staphylococcus aureus*; NA, narcotics anonymous; PPD, purified protein derivative; PFT, pulmonary function test; PTSD, posttraumatic stress disorder; SI, suicidal ideation; TB, tuberculosis; TSH, thyroid-stimulating hormone; UA, urinalysis.

TABLE 3-35 Assessment of Treatment Readiness with the Stages of Change Model

Stage of Change	Perspective on Change
1. Precontemplation	No problem observed, no intent to change
2. Contemplation	Problem observed, ambivalent about change
3. Preparation	Problem acknowledged; patient preparing to change
4. Action	Change initiated to correct problem
5. Maintenance	Sustained change to correct problem
6. Relapse	Recurrence of problematic behavior and ambivalence about or denial of problem

Adapted from Prochaska JO, DiClemente CC. Stages and processes of self-change of smoking: toward an integrative model of change. *J Consult Clin Psychol* 1983;51(3): 390–395.

General Treatment Principles

- The choice of treatment method should be tailored to the individual and should include:
  - Psychosocial treatments (including counseling and other behavioral therapies, self-help groups)
  - Treatment of co-occurring psychiatric disorders. There is no specified timeline for defining co-occurring Axis I disorders, but clinical consensus is after 4 weeks of abstinence
  - Medications, including abstinence maintenance therapy
- Detoxification alone does not change long-term use patterns
- Sustained reduction in the use and improvement of associated psychiatric symptoms is much more likely after treatment of at least 3 months
- The outcome or efficacy of treatment is very dependent on the skills of individual counselors
- Monitor often for drug use during treatment. Urine toxicology or Breathalyzer screens are often helpful adjuncts to treatment for achieving and maintaining abstinence
- Evaluate for infectious diseases, including HIV/AIDS, hepatitis B and C, and tuberculosis, and counsel the patient on modification of risky behaviors
- Recovery often requires multiple episodes of treatment

Unexplained Medical Symptoms

Syndromes of unexplained medical symptoms are characterized by bodily complaints that suggest a physical disorder but for which no organic or physiologic cause can be found. These patients view their symptoms as physical in origin and present to primary care or specialty clinics. Psychiatrists are most frequently consulted for help when the primary team has determined that the symptoms are not "real." It may be necessary to differentiate between the various subcategories of somatoform disorders and factitious disorder and malingering, as described below.

TABLE 3-36 Differential Diagnosis of Unexplained Medical Symptoms

Nonpsychiatric Conditions	Psychiatric Conditions
Organic disease: rule out first Functional medical syndromes: • Irritable bowel syndrome • Chronic fatigue syndrome • Fibromyalgia • Pain syndrome	Somatoform disorders • Depression • Anxiety or panic • OCD • Psychosis • Factitious disorder • Malingering

OCD, obsessive–compulsive disorder.

TABLE 3-37 Evaluation of Somatoform Disorders

History with special attention to:

History of present illness:

- Histories are often vague, inconsistent, and imprecise; chronologies are disorganized.
- Consider asking patients to graph symptom severity vs. time; important events, such as surgery, may be added in
- Symptom presentation is often "atypical," but patients are suggestible and may learn a more typical presentation
- The idea of a psychogenic etiology is often unacceptable to patients, who describe their symptoms in purely physical terms
- "La belle indifference": a seeming lack of concern about debilitating symptoms; has been sited as a sign of somatization but is not helpful in ruling out organic illness (i.e., acute stroke)

Psychiatric history: comorbid psychiatric diagnoses are common, particularly mood or anxiety disorders; assess history of trauma or abuse
Medications: current medications and compliance
Family history: history of parental illness during the patient's childhood
Social history: extent of functional impairment with regarding job and relationships
Review of systems: typically diffusely positive; attempting to obtain details may be fruitless and time consuming
Medical history: be sure to obtain records from past providers and, other hospitals; patients may have voluminous charts showing large numbers of futile examinations, surgery, and medical attempts at treatment; there may be a history of mutual hostility between patients and doctors, resulting in doctor shopping

General Medical and Neurologic Examination with special attention to:

- Assess signs of organic disease
- A good physical examination may be therapeutic and reassuring to the patient
- Pay special attention to scars and other signs of past medical intervention
- Avoid attempts to trick the patient (e.g., the "touch/no touch" or "arm-drop" tests during the neurologic examination) because results are often nonspecific and trickery may damage the therapeutic relationship

Psychiatric Mental Status Examination

Laboratory Studies, Imaging, and Other Diagnostic Tools

Usually not indicated; avoid unnecessary investigations

SOMATOFORM DISORDERS

Somatization Disorder and Undifferentiated Somatoform Disorders

- Chronic syndromes of recurring multiple somatic symptoms that are not medically explainable
- The *DSM-IV* requires four pain, two gastrointestinal, one sexual, and one pseudoneurologic symptoms for diagnosis
- Symptoms are associated with psychosocial distress (including diagnoses of depression and anxiety) and medical help seeking
- Typical onset is before age 30 years
- Prevalence is between 1% and 2% of community and primary care samples
- It is twice as common in women as in men
- Risk factors include:
  - History of physical or sexual abuse
  - Parental illness
  - Unexplained somatic symptoms in childhood
  - Nonwhite race, low income, less education

Conversion or Dissociation Disorder ("hysteria")

- Pseudoneurologic symptoms (e.g., paralysis, blindness, amnesia, seizure) of sudden onset that closely follow a traumatic event or significant life stressor
- The conditions are not based on "real" disease but rather on how patients believe their bodies can fail them (e.g., a patient cannot talk above a whisper but can produce a loud cough)
- There is a good prognosis for acute conversion but a relatively poor one for longer lasting symptoms
- There may be an increased risk of suicide among female patients

Hypochondriasis

- Characterized by a triad of disease conviction, functional impairment, and refusal to accept appropriate reassurance (i.e., an overvalued morbid preoccupation with one's body)
- The *DSM-IV* diagnosis of hypochondriasis cannot be made if symptoms are better explained by major depression, panic disorder, or generalized anxiety disorder. For example:
  - Illness phobia: patients are afraid of illnesses they have yet to encounter; hypochondriasis: patients are convinced they are already sick
  - Panic disorder: patients fear that they are imminently dying; hypochondriasis: patients fear long-term consequences of occult illness
- Prevalence varies according to the strictness of definition (0.8%–5%)
- The prevalence is similar in men and women, and the prevalence does not vary significantly with age. Patients who have had serious childhood illness are at higher risk
- A chronic, fluctuating course that is influenced by stressful circumstances may be seen

Body Dysmorphic Disorder

- A distressing preoccupation with a nonexistent or slight defect in appearance along with the belief that one is defective and unappealing
- It may involve any part of the body, but the face, skin, and genitals are most common. Bodily asymmetry and overall appearance are also common
- Preoccupations are time consuming and difficult to control and result in social impairment
- Patients may be delusional or believe others are staring at or mocking their "defect"
- More than 90% of patients perform time-consuming behaviors to correct the defect, hide it, or paradoxically convince others of its ugliness
- Common comorbidities include major depression, social phobia, substance-related disorders, and OCD
- SSRIs are often helpful in treatment
- The prevalence is similar in men and women

Principles of Management

- Establish a therapeutic alliance with patients by acknowledging the reality of their symptoms and their suffering despite the absence of "disease"
- Avoid unnecessary pharmacologic treatment, investigations, procedures, and hospitalizations ("First, do no harm")
- Manage expectations; the goal is to help patients deal with their symptoms, not necessarily to cure them
- Patients may benefit from "face-saving" opportunities to resolve their symptoms (e.g., physical therapy or being told that response to a given intervention will distinguish physical from functional syndromes)
- Treat comorbid conditions. The most commonly missed concurrent conditions are psychiatric (usually mood or anxiety disorders)
- According to a 2007 meta-analysis by Kroenke, CBT is consistently helpful across a spectrum of somatoform disorders
- Likewise, preliminary evidence suggests that antidepressants are helpful, even in the absence of a mood disorder
- Patients in treatment with a primary care physician (PCP) may benefit from a psychiatric consult letter to the PCP outlining the principles of treatment, such as making frequent, brief appointments

MALINGERING AND FACTITIOUS DISORDER

Patients with somatoform disorders are not conscious of the mechanism of their symptom production. They are not "faking," and they cannot control their symptoms. Malingering and factitious disorder, in contrast, are often termed "syndromes of voluntary symptom production," implying both control and volition. However, patients with factitious disorder are clearly ill, and the term "voluntary," with the blame that is assigns, should be used with caution.

Malingering

- The patient fabricates or exaggerates the symptoms of a mental or physical disorder to reach an obvious goal or purpose (i.e., avoid criminal prosecution, obtain pain medication)
- Suspect malingering if any of the following is present:
  - A medicolegal context
  - A marked discrepancy between the ostensible distress or disability and the objective findings
  - A lack of cooperation with the diagnostic evaluation or treatment regimen
  - The presence of antisocial personality disorder
- In appropriate circumstances, the patient should be informed that failure to comply with evaluation or treatment will be seen as evidence of malingering (i.e., when he or she is seeking disability insurance or pain medication)

Factitious Disorder

- Patients simulate or feign disease, with the primary motivation of assuming the sick role
- There is no obvious advantage to the factitious illness; in fact, patients may put their health at considerable risk
- There may be little or no insight into the reasons for the self-destructive behavior
- Presentation may include psychological symptoms (i.e., factitious bereavement for a person who does not exist), physical symptoms, or a combination of both
- The category includes factitious disorder by proxy
- Patients show considerable ingenuity in feigning illness; some common strategies include:
  - Factitious fever by warming thermometers
  - Production of real fever and infection by injected infected material (sputum, feces, tuberculosis and other organisms) into skin or veins
  - Tampering with prior wounds or surgical scars to prevent healing
  - Feigning of hematologic disorders by surreptitious self-administration of warfarin or heparin
  - Factitious hypoglycemia by injection of insulin (check C peptide levels)

Demographics

- Rare (0.4%–0.8% of all psychiatric consultations) but possibly underdiagnosed
- Typically begins before age 30 years
- Associated with high rates of substance abuse, mood disorder, and borderline personality disorder

Treatment and Management

- Factitious disorder tends to be chronic
- Engaging a patient with factitious disorder in long-term psychiatric treatment is extremely rare

- **Confrontational approach to management:**
  - Confront the patient with tangible evidence of fabrication
  - Be nonpunitive and supportive
  - Stress continuity of care
  - Emphasize that the patient is sick and needs help
- **Nonconfrontational approach:**
  - Give the patient a "face-saving" option, such as the therapeutic double-bind (if this symptoms does not improve after this procedure, it will mean that it is factitious)
- The psychiatrist may be helpful in organizing a meeting at which staff can vent and express the anger that frequently accompanies the diagnosis of factitious disorder

REFERENCES

ANXIETY

American Psychiatric Association. *Diagnostic and Statistical Manual of Mental Disorders*, ed 4, text rev. Washington, DC: American Psychiatric Association; 2000.

Iosifescu D, Pollack M. An approach to the anxious patient: symptoms of anxiety, fear, avoidance, or increased arousal. In Stern TA (d.). *The Ten-Minute Guide to Psychiatric Diagnosis and Treatment.* New York: Professional Publishing; 2005:197–224.

Katon W. Panic disorder. *N Engl J Med* 2006;354:2360–2367.

Sadock BJ, Sadock VA (eds). *Kaplan and Sadock's Synopsis of Psychiatry.* Philadelphia: Lippincott Williams & Wilkins; 2003.

DEMENTIA

Stern TA, Herman JB, Slavin PL. *The Massachusetts General Hospital Guide to Primary Care Psychiatry,* 5th ed. 2004:198.

DEPRESSION

American Psychiatric Association. *Quick Reference to the Diagnostic Criteria from DSM-IV-TR.* Arlington, VA: American Psychiatric Association; 2000.

Goldberg RJ. *The Care of the Psychiatric Patient,* 2nd ed. Mosby, Inc. 1998.

Sadock BJ, Sadock VA (eds). *Kaplan and Sadock's Synopsis of Psychiatry.* Philadelphia: Lippincott Williams & Wilkins; 2003.

Rosenbaum JF, Arana GW, Hyman SE, et al. *Handbook of Psychiatric Drug Therapy,* 5th ed. Philadelphia: Lippincott Williams & Wilkins; 2005.

DISORDERED EATING BEHAVIORS

American Psychiatric Association. *Diagnostic and Statistical Manual of Mental Disorders,* ed 4, text rev. Washington, DC: American Psychiatric Association; 2000.

Sadock BJ, Sadock VA (eds). *Kaplan and Sadock's Synopsis of Psychiatry.* Philadelphia: Lippincott Williams & Wilkins; 2003.

DISSOCIATION

Chu JA. Rebuilding shattered lives. In *The Responsible Treatment of Complex Posttraumatic and Dissociative Disorders.* New York: John Wiley & Sons; 1998.

Howell EF. *The Dissociative Mind.* New York: The Analytic Press; 2005.

Keane TM, Kaufman ML, Kimble MO. Peritraumatic dissociative symptoms, acute stress disorder, and the development of posttraumatic stress disorder: causation, correlation or epiphenomenon? In Sanchez-Planell L, Diez-Quevedo C (eds). *Dissociative States.* New York: Springer Verlag; 2000:21–43.

Lowenstein RA. An office mental status examination for complex chronic dissociative symptoms and multiple personality disorder. *Psychiatr Clin North Am* 1991;14: 567–604.

Simeone D, Knutelska M, Nelson D, et al. Feeling unreal: a depersonalization disorder update of 117 cases. *J Clin Psychiatry* 2003;64:990–997.

Steinberg M, Schnall M. *The Stranger in the Mirror: Dissociation: The Hidden Epidemic.* New York: Harper Collins; 2000.

MANIA

Diagnostic and Statistical Manual of Mental Disorders, 4th edition, text revision, 2000. Arlington, VA: American Psychiatric Association.

Hirschfeld RM, Bowden CL, Gitlin MJ, Keck PE, Suppes T, Thase ME, Wagner KD, Perlis RH, 2002. Practice guideline for the treatment of patients with bipolar disorder. Arlington, VA; American Psychiatric Association. Available at http://www.psych.org/psych_pract/treatg/pg/prac_guide.cfm.

Muller-Oerlinghausen B, Bereghofer A, Bauer M. Bipolar Disorder. *Lancet* 2002;359: 241–7.

Sadock BJ, Sadock VA. *Kaplan and Sadock's Synopsis of Psychiatry.* Philadelphia: Lippincott Williams & Wilkins, 2003.

OBSESSIONS AND COMPULSIONS

Sadock BJ, Sadock V (eds). *Kaplan and Sadock's Synopsis of Psychiatry.* Philadelphia: Lippincott Williams & Wilkins; 2003:616–623.

Simson HB, Foa EB, Liebowitz MR, et al. A randomized, controlled trial of cognitive-behavioral therapy for augmenting pharmacotherapy in obsessive-compulsive disorder. *Am J Psychiatry* 2008;165(5):621–630.

PERSONALITY DISORDERS

American Psychiatric Association. *Diagnostic and Statistical Manual of Mental Disorders,* ed 4, text rev. Washington, DC: American Psychiatric Association; 2000.

Leichsenring F, Leibing E. The effectiveness of psychodynamic therapy and cognitive behavior therapy in the treatment of personality disorders: a meta-analysis. *Am J Psychiatry* 2004;160:1223–1232.

O'Donahue W, Fowler AK, Lilienfeld SO. *Personality Disorders—Toward the DSM-V.* Los Angeles: Sage Publications; 2007.

Oldham JM, Skodol AE, Bender DS. *Textbook of Personality Disorders.* Washington, DC: American Psychiatric Publishing; 2005.

Perry JC, Banon E, Ianni F. Effectiveness of psychotherapy for personality disorders. *Am J Psychiatry* 1999;156:1312–1321.

Sadock BJ, Sadock VA (eds). *Kaplan and Sadock's Synopsis of Psychiatry.* Philadelphia: Lippincott Williams & Wilkins; 2003.

PROBLEMS WITH SEXUAL FUNCTION AND BEHAVIORS

Sadock BJ, Sadock VA (eds). Human sexuality & gender identity disorders. In *Kaplan and Sadock's Synopsis of Psychiatry,* 9th ed. Philadelphia: Lippincott Williams & Wilkins; 2003:692–738.

Saleh FM, Berlin FS, Malin HM, et al. Paraphilias and paraphilia-like disorders. In *Gabbard's Treatments of Psychiatric Disorders,* 4th ed. Washington, DC: American Psychiatric Publishing; 2007:671–682.

Shafer L. Sexual Disorders and sexual dysfunction. In *Massachusetts General Hospital Psychiatry Update & Board Preparation,* 2nd ed. New York: McGraw-Hill; 2004: 155–164.

PSYCHOSIS

Azorin JM, Akiskal H, Akiskal K, et al. Is psychosis in DSMIV mania due to severity? The relevance of selected demographic and comorbid social-phobic features. *Acta Psychiatr Scand* 2007;115:29–34.

Ciapparelli A, Paggini R, Marazziti D, et al. Comorbidity with axis I anxiety disorders in remitted psychotic patients 1 year after hospitalization. *CNS Spect* 2007;12:913–919.

Freudenreich O, Holt DJ, Cather C, et al. The evaluation and management of patients with first-episode schizophrenia: a selective, clinical review of diagnosis, treatment, and prognosis. *Harvard Rev Psychiatry* 2007;15:189–211.

Jibson MD. Overview of psychosis. In Rose BD (ed). *UpToDate.* Waltham, MA; 2007.

Kane J. Clinical efficacy of clozapine in treatment of refractory schizophrenia: an overview. *Br J Psychiatry* 1992;18:41–54.

McEvoy JP, Lieberman JA, Perkins DO, et al. Efficacy and tolerability of olanzapine, quetiapine, and risperidone in the treatment of early psychosis: a randomized, double-blind 52-week comparison. *Am J Psychiatry* 2007;164:1050–1060.

Motlová L, Španiel F, Höschl C, et al. Are there any differences in the efficacy among second generation antipsychotics in the treatment of schizophrenia and related disorders? *Ann Clin Psychiatry* 2007;19:133–143.

Perala J, Suvisaari J, Saarni SI, et al. Lifetime prevalence of psychotic and bipolar I disorders in a general population. *Arch Gen Psychiatry* 2007;64:19–28.

Peralta V, Cuesta MJ. Diagnostic significance of Schneider's first-rank symptoms in schizophrenia. Comparative study between schizophrenic and non-schizophrenic psychotic disorders. *Br J Psychiatry* 1999;174:243–248.

Rosenbaum JF, Arana GW, Hyman SE, et al:. *Handbook of Psychiatric Drug Therapy*, 5th ed. Philadelphia: Lippincott Williams & Wilkins; 2005.

Sadock BJ, Sadock VA (eds). *Kaplan & Sadock's Comprehensive Textbook of Psychiatry*, 8th ed. Philadelphia: Lippincott Williams & Wilkins; 2004.

Sadock BJ, Sadock VA (eds). *Kaplan & Sadock's Pocket Handbook of Clinical Psychiatry*, 4th ed. Philadelphia: Lippincott Williams & Wilkins; 2005.

Stern TA, Herman JB (eds). *Massachusetts General Hospital Psychiatry Update & Board Preparation*, 2nd ed. New York: McGraw Hill; 2003.

Strahl NR. *Clinical Study Guide for the Oral Boards in Psychiatry*, 2nd ed. Washington DC: American Psychiatric Publishing; 2005.

Stroup TS, McEvoy JP, Swartz MS, et al. The National Institute of Mental Health Clinical Antipsychotic Trials of Intervention Effectiveness (CATIE) project: schizophrenia trial design and protocol development. *Schizophr Bull* 2003;29:15–31.

Vieweg WV. New generation antipsychotic drugs and QTc interval prolongation. *Prim Care Companion J Clin Psychiatry* 2003;5:205–215.

SLEEP DISORDERS

Basner RC. Continuous positive airway pressure for obstructive sleep apnea. *N Engl J Med* 2007;356:1751–1758.

Buysse DJ, Germain A, Moul D, et al. Insomnia. In Buysse DJ (ed). *Sleep Disorders and Psychiatry.* Washington, DC: American Psychiatric Publishing; 2005:29–75.

Eckert DJ, Jordan AS, Merchia P, et al. Central sleep apnea: pathophysiology and treatment. *Chest* 2007;131:595–607.

Fahey CD, Zee PC. Circadian rhythm sleep disorders and phototherapy. *Psychiatr Clin North Am* 2006;29:989–1007.

Nishino S. Narcolepsy: pathophysiology and pharmacology. *J Clin Psychiatry* 2007; 68(suppl 13):9–15.

Plante DT, Winkelman JW. Parasomnias. *Psychiatr Clin North Am* 2006;29:969–987.

Winkelman JW. Restless legs syndrome. In Buysse DJ (ed). *Sleep Disorders and Psychiatry.* Washington, DC: American Psychiatric Publishing; 2005:139–162.

Young TJ, Silber MH. Hypersomnias of central origin. *Chest* 2006;130(3):913–920.

SUBSTANCE USE DISORDERS

Centers for Disease Control and Prevention. *Suicide Facts At A Glance. Data Sheet*; Summer 2007. Available at: http://www.cdc.gov/ncipc/dvp/Suicide/SuicideDataSheet.pdf.

Comptom WM, Thomas YF, Stinson FS, et al. Prevalence, correlates, disability, and comorbidity of DSM-IV drug abuse and dependence in the United States: results from the national epidemiologic survey on alcohol and related conditions. *Arch Gen Psychiatry* 2007;64:566–576.

Hettema J, Steele J, Miller WR. Motivational interviewing. *Ann Rev Clin Psychol* 2005;1:91–111.

Mersy D. Recognition of alcohol and substance abuse. *Am Fam Physician* 2003;67(7): 1529–1532.

National Institute of Drug Abuse and the National Institutes of Health. *Principles of Drug Addiction Treatment: A Research-Based Guide.* Available at: http://www.nida.nih.gov/PODAT/PODAT8.html.

National Institutes of Health. *Fact Sheet: Addiction and the Criminal Justice System.* Available at: http://www.nih.gov/about/researchresultsforthepublic/addiction.pdf.

Nunes EV, Rousaville BJ. Co-morbidity of substance use with depression and other mental disorders: from Diagnostic and Statistical Manual of Mental Disorders, fourth edition (DSM-IV) to DSV-V. Research report. *Addiction* 2006;101(suppl 1):89–96.

Prochaska JO, DiClemente CC. Stages and processes of self-change of smoking: toward an integrative model of change. *J Consult Clin Psychol* 1983;51(3) 390–395.

Regier DA, Farmer ME, Rae DS, et al. Comorbidity of mental disorders with alcohol and other drug abuse: results from the Epidemiologic Catchment Area (ECA) study. *JAMA* 1990;262:2511–2518.

Rollnick S, Miller WR. What is motivational interviewing? *Behav Cognitive Psychother* 1995;23:325–334.

Sadock BJ, Sadock VA (eds). *Kaplan & Sadock's Synopsis of Psychiatry*, 9th ed. Philadelphia: Lippincott Williams & Wilkins; 2003:380–470.

Substance Abuse and Mental Health Services Administration. *Results from the 2006 National Survey on Drug Use and Health: National Findings.* NSDUH Series H-32, DHHS Publication No. SMA 07-4293. Rockville, MD: Office of Applied Studies; 2007. Available at: http://oas.samhsa.gov/nsduh/2k6nsduh/2k6Results.cfm#Ch7.

Weaver MF, Jarvis MA, Gold MS, et al. Overview of the recognition and management of the drug abuser. In Basow DS (ed). *UpToDate.* Waltham, MA: Wolters Kluwer; 2008.

UNEXPLAINED MEDICAL SYMPTOMS

Cassem NH, Sterm TA, Rosebaum JF (eds). *Massachusetts General Hospital Handbook of General Hospital Psychiatry.* St. Louis: Mosby Year Book; 1997.

Gelder MG, Lopez-Ibor JJ, Andreasen N (eds). *New Oxford Textbook of Psychiatry.* UK: Oxford University Press; 2001.

Kendell R, Jablensky A. Distinguishing between the validity and utility of psychiatric diagnoses. *Am J Psychiatry* 2003;160:4–12.

Kroenke K. Efficacy of treatment for somatoform disorders: a review of randomized controlled trials. *Psychosom Med* 2007;69:881–888.

Noyes R Jr, Stuart SP, Watson DB. A reconceptualization of somatoform disorders. *Psyhosomatics* 2008;49:114–122.

Chapter 4

SPECIAL POPULATIONS

Children and Adolescents

The psychiatric evaluation of children differs from that of adults in several key ways. Clinicians must take into consideration:

- The developmental stage of the child
- Agitation: etiology and management
- Legal obligations: role of the legal guardian, mandatory reporting of suspected abuse or neglect
- Somatic complaints are common presentations; a high suspicion for underlying medical conditions and developmental delays must be maintained
- Role of family and school: children often present because of behavioral dyscontrol at home or school or because of social or family crises. Family and school are also critical to include in the treatment plan

TABLE 4-1 Approach to the Evaluation of Children and Adolescents

History and Physical Examination
Before you begin: • Determine who has legal custody of the child and obtain consent for evaluation (see below) • Determine the developmental age of the child and the appropriate interview technique **History:** • Sources: patient, family, caregivers, treaters, teachers • Assess for Axis I and II disorders with special attention to somatic symptoms, eating patterns, level of functioning (school, social, family), self-destructive behavior (suicide, dangerous or reckless behavior, substance abuse, cutting or burning) **Medical history:** • Perinatal history: full-term, prenatal exposure to toxins or alcohol, perinatal complications • Developmental history: milestones, previous occupational or speech therapy • General: history of seizures, trauma, recurrent ear infections **Social history:** • Grade in school; who lives in the home; adult and peer supports; school performance, including special education or individualized education programs (IEP); friends; social activities; sports; hobbies; screen time • Department of Social Services involvement, legal or court involvement • Abuse history: physical, sexual, bullying, verbal, neglect **Physical examination:** • Special attention to growth and development, signs of injury or trauma, nutritional status, dysmorphic features

(continued)

TABLE 4-1 Approach to the Evaluation of Children and Adolescents (*continued*)

Psychiatric Mental Status Examination with special attention to:
• Eye contact, motor activity, presence of verbal or motor tics, stuttering, vocabulary, developmental stage • Additional approaches: ask the child to draw a picture of his or her family (assess fine motor skills and attention); ask the child for "three wishes" (assesses child's projective and future-oriented thinking) • Observe interactions between the guardian and child
Laboratory Studies, Imaging, and Other Diagnostic Tools
First-line studies: β-HCG, urine toxicology (blood draws rarely indicated) **Second-line studies, if indicated:** serum toxicology, electrolytes, blood levels of medications, EKG, EEG, CT

CT, computed tomography; EEG, electroencephalography; EKG, electrocardiography; HCG, human chorionic gonadotropin

TABLE 4-2 Developmental Milestones

Developmental Milestones (Normal Age)		
Motor	**Language**	**Adaptive**
Rolls front and back (4 mo)	Smiling (4–6 wks)	Mouthing (3 mo)
Sits with support (6 mo)	Coos (3 mo)	Transfers objects (6 mo)
Sits alone (9–10 mo)	Babbles (6 mo)	Picks up raisin (11–12 mo)
Pulls to stand (10 mo)	Uses jargon (10–14 mo)	Scribbles (15 mo)
Crawls (10–12 mo)	Speaks first word (12 mo)	Drinks from cup (10 mo)
Walks alone (10–18 mo)	Follows one-step commands (15 mo)	Uses spoon (12–15 mo)
Runs (15–24 mo)	Follows two- word combination (22 mo)	Bladder trained (<5 yo)
Rides a tricycle (3 yrs)	Follows three-word sentences (3 yr)	Bowel train (<4 yo)
Rides a bicycle (5–7 yrs)		

Psychiatric Emergencies in Children and Adolescents

Agitation

About 25% of adolescent emergency psychiatric evaluations are because of aggressive behavior.

MANAGEMENT OF THE AGITATED CHILD

Behavioral Management

- Speak and approach the child in a calm, reassuring manner
- Ask a family member to stay with the child if his or her presence is calming or soothing
- Offer a drink, snack, or toys if available
- Provide a time-out in a room with little stimulation (*continued*)

TABLE 4-3 Differential Diagnosis of the Agitated Child

Nonpsychiatric Conditions

Metabolic and systemic disorders: poisoning or exposure to toxin, acute infection
Neurologic disorders: delirium, meningitis, space-occupying lesion, seizure, acute confusional migraine, head trauma
Medications: corticosteroids, bronchodilators

Psychiatric Conditions

- Psychosis
- Mania
- Severe anxiety
- Acute stress disorder
- PTSD
- Substances: intoxication or withdrawal
- ADHD
- Conduct disorder
- developmental delay

ADHD, attention-deficit hyperactivity disorder; ODD, oppositional defiant disorder; PTSD, posttraumatic stress disorder.

(continued)

Pharmacologic Management

- A clinician requires permission from parent or guardian to administer nonemergency medication
- Use as-needed (PRN) medications or an additional dose of the child's standing medication if available
- Diphenhydramine: 1.25 mg/kg/dose orally (PO) or intramuscularly (IM) (check that the child has no history of paradoxical excitation with this medication)
- Clonidine: 0.05 mg–0.1 mg PO depending on the child's age and size
- Risperidone: 0.5–1.0 mg PO depending on the child's age and size
- If child with acute agitation is older than 16 years of age:
  - Haloperidol: 2.5–5.0 mg PO or IM
  - Plus lorazepam: 1 mg PO or IM
  - Plus diphenhydramine: 50 mg PO or IM

Seclusion and Restraints

- Use if the child is in imminent danger of harming him- or herself or others
- Ask the family to leave the room
- Follow Department of Health observation protocols

Suicide

- Suicide is the third leading cause of death in people aged 10 to 24 years
- In 2005, 16.9% of adolescents had considered suicide, and 8.4% had attempted suicide within the past year. Firearms are most common method for boys and young men
- See page 35 for suicide assessment and management

Abuse and Neglect

- Mandatory reporting of suspected child abuse:
  - Report any suspected child abuse or neglect to Child Protective Services or the Department of Social Services
  - Keeping the child safe is first priority. Consider admitting the child to the hospital

Psychiatric Symptoms Caused by a Medical Condition in Pediatric Patients

TABLE 4-4 Psychiatric Symptoms Caused by a Medical Condition in Pediatric Patients

Depression	
• Malignancy • Hypothyroidism • Anemia • SLE • AIDS	• Diabetes • Epilepsy • Medications (stimulants, neuroleptics, corticosteroids, contraceptives)
Anxiety	
• Hyperthyroidism • Cardiac arrhythmia • Pheochromocytoma • Migraine	• Marfan syndrome • High caffeine intake • Stimulant use, including nicotine • Adverse medication reaction
OCD	
• Carbon monoxide poisoning • PANDAS • Postviral encephalitis	• Prader-Willi syndrome • Sydenham's chorea • TBI
Psychosis	
• Delirium • Seizure • Intoxication or withdrawal • CNS lesion (tumors, trauma, congenital malformation)	• Developmental disorder (e.g., velocardiofacial syndrome) • Neurologic disease (Wilson's disease, toxic encephalopathy) • Infectious disease (encephalitis, meningitis, HIV)
Mania	
• MS • Temporal lobe seizure • Intoxication • Kleine-Levin syndrome	• Hyperthyroidism • Uremia • Wilson's disease • Porphyria

CNS, central nervous system; HIV, human immunodeficiency virus; MS, multiple sclerosis; OCD, obsessive–compulsive disorder; PANDAS, pediatric autoimmune disorder associated with *Streptococcal* infection; SLE, systemic lupus erythematosus; TBI, traumatic brain injury. Adapted from Guerrero AP: General medical considerations in child and adolescent patients who present with psychiatric symptoms. *Child Adolesc Psychiatr Clin N Am* 2003;12:613–628.

Potential Causes of Behavioral Problems in Children and Adolescents

- Normal oppositional behavior for developmental stage (shorter duration, less frequent, less intense)
- Cognitive disorder or learning disorders
- Oppositional defiant disorder (ODD)

- Conduct disorder
- Adjustment disorder (shorter duration, linked to stressor)
- Psychotic disorders
- Mood disorders
- Attention-deficit hyperactivity disorder (ADHD)
- Substance abuse
- Obsessive–compulsive disorder (OCD)
- Medical illness

SELECTED DISORDERS IN CHILD AND ADOLESCENT PSYCHIATRY

Pervasive Developmental Disorders (PDDs)

- **Definition:** a group of disorders presenting in early childhood characterized by impaired language or communication, socialization, and stereotyped behaviors
- Includes autism, Rett's disorder, childhood disintegrative disorder, Asperger's disorder, and PDD not otherwise specified (NOS)
- Can be associated with mental retardation, genetic abnormalities, congenital infections, and other medical conditions

Autism

- Significant and sustained impairment in social interaction and communication with stereotyped behaviors
- Prevalence is about 1 in 1,000 children. The prevalence of autism spectrum disorders is between 1 in 150 and 1 in 500. The male-to-female ratio is 4 to 1
- **Treatment:**
  - Early intervention should include therapy and a focus on social interaction
  - Antipsychotics can be helpful for behavioral disturbances, stimulants for inattention, and selective serotonin reuptake inhibitors (SSRIs) for co-occurring mood or anxiety disorders
  - Risperidone is approved for treatment of irritability and aggression in children with autism

Attention-Deficit Hyperactivity Disorder

- Maladaptive pattern of clinically significant inattention, hyperactivity, or impulsivity
- Begins before age 7 years and may persist into adulthood
- Symptoms may not be apparent in a structured clinic setting but must be apparent in more than one setting (e.g., school and home)
- Prevalence estimates vary between 2% and 16%. The male-to-female ratio is 4 to 1 for predominantly hyperactive type and 2 to 1 for predominantly inattentive type
- The differential diagnosis of nonpsychiatric causes includes vision or hearing impairment, seizures, head trauma, malnutrition, and sleep disturbance

Treatment

- Stimulants are first-line therapy. Caution should be used in children with history of seizures, Tourette's disease, PDD, substance abusers in the household, and age younger than 6 years
- Consider the use of clonidine and guanfacine in young children
- Atomoxetine is an alternate first-line choice in school-aged children. Second-line treatments include tricyclic antidepressants (TCAs), bupropion, clonidine, and guanfacine hydrochloride
- Investigational drugs include modafinil, tacrine, and donepezil
- Behavioral strategies include an increased structure and rewarding positive behavior

WHEN TO REFER TO A CHILD PSYCHIATRIST

- Age younger than 6 years at presentation
- Comorbid psychiatric, neurologic, or medical conditions
- Lack of response to initial treatment with stimulant or atomoxetine

Substance Abuse

- Common among teenagers. In 2007, 20% of 12th graders and 7% of 8th graders had used an illicit drug in the past month
- Most commonly abused substances in teens: alcohol > tobacco > marijuana > inhalants > opiates > cocaine > hallucinogens > tranquilizers > methamphetamine, anabolic steroids, and cough medicine
- Risk factors for substance abuse in adolescents: aggression or impulsivity, alienation from parents, experimentation before age 15 years, family violence, homelessness, low self-esteem, physical or sexual abuse, poor social integration, posttraumatic stress disorder (PTSD), rebelliousness, relationship with peers who have substance use issues

Legal Issues in the Psychiatric Care of Children

- Minors (children younger than 18 years of age) are presumed to lack the capacity to consent for medical care
- Emancipated minors are youths younger than age 18 years who are married, pregnant, have children, or are determined by the court to be self-sufficient
- If the patient is a minor:
  - Determine who the legal guardian is
  - The legal guardian must be physically present in the emergency room except in the case of emergency stabilization
  - Legal guardians must consent to outpatient and inpatient treatment
  - If necessary, consult with an attorney or hospital legal office and familiarize yourself with the laws of your particular state

Women

- Women are prone to relapse of existing psychiatric illness and initial presentation of psychiatric illness during times of reproductive transition (e.g., menstruation, pregnancy, and the postpartum period)

- Treatment of psychiatric illness in women must take into consideration reproductive safety

Differences in the Prevalence and Presentation of Psychiatric Illness in Women

- Major depression: 25% among women (vs. 10% in the general population)
- Panic disorder, eating disorders, and some personality disorders are more prevalent in women
- Schizophrenia onset is 5 to 10 years later in women; it is also more apt to occur in the perimenopausal period
- Women are more likely to attempt suicide and less likely to use lethal means

Pregnancy

- About 20% of women may experience mood or anxiety disorders during pregnancy
- Pregnancy is *not* protective for relapse or initial presentation of psychiatric disorders
- Maintenance treatment for psychiatric illnesses may be indicated to prevent relapse or exacerbation during pregnancy and the postpartum period
- The postpartum period (≤6 months after delivery) is a high-risk period for the emergence or reemergence of Axis I disorders
- Women are at increased risk for domestic violence while they are pregnant; screening for violence is advised
- Assess for the well-being of the infant; reporting to local child services agency is mandated if abuse or neglect are suspected

Postpartum Illness

POSTPARTUM BLUES

- **Definition:** a common, mild mood disturbance in the immediate postpartum period
- **Onset:** occurs in up to 75% of postpartum women. Symptoms generally peak 4 days after delivery and resolve within 2 weeks
- **Presentation:** mood symptoms are transient; joy is interspersed with sadness or mood lability, anxiety, and tearfulness; neurovegetative symptoms, anhedonia, or suicidal ideation (SI) are rare
- **Treatment:** reassurance, support with practical activities for the baby's care
- If present for more 2 weeks, depression may be diagnosed

POSTPARTUM DEPRESSION

- **Definition:** a depressive episode that occurs in the postpartum period
- **Onset:** typically between 4 weeks and 12 months postpartum; may emerge at any time after delivery
- **Presentation:** manifested by symptoms of major depression; depressive and anxious ruminations predominate; may include thoughts of harming the baby, typically without a plan, that are upsetting to the mother
- **Incidence:** 10% to 20% of postpartum women

- **Risk factors:** history of postpartum depression, prior depressive disorder (including bipolar disorder), depression during pregnancy, neonatal complications, poor social supports, high stressors
- **Treatment:** antidepressants, reassurance, ongoing safety evaluation (of both the mother and child)
- May occur with any pregnancy loss (including miscarriage and abortion)

POSTPARTUM PSYCHOSIS

- **Definition:** a psychotic episode during the postpartum period
- **Onset:** any time; the majority develop within first 2 weeks after delivery; often emerges rapidly as part of manic or mixed episode
- **Presentation:** typically paranoia, delusions of guilt and sin, or delusions centering on the infant; may have command hallucinations to harm the baby
    - May present as grossly disorganized thinking
    - Associated with insomnia, restlessness, and irritability
    - Increased risk of infanticide or suicide
- **Incidence:** 0.1% to 0.2% of postpartum women
- **Risk factors:** bipolar disorder (30% association), previous history of postpartum psychosis or depression
- **Treatment:** inpatient treatment, antipsychotics, antidepressants, safe child custody and care

Psychopharmacologic Treatment During Pregnancy and the Postpartum Period

GENERAL PRINCIPLES

- Psychiatric illnesses carry risks for both the mother and fetus if left untreated
- Medications are typically class C (e.g., "risk cannot be ruled out")
- Although many medications have available data to support first trimester safety, knowledge of prenatal exposure is incomplete
- The three classes of risk are teratogenesis, neonatal toxicity, and long-term neuropsychiatric consequences
- Reproductive safety should be discussed with *every* woman of reproductive age, regardless of her plans for pregnancy

ANTIDEPRESSANTS

- SSRIs are generally considered safe to use during pregnancy, with some exceptions:
    - The most data exist for fluoxetine, showing no increased risk of congenital malformation
    - Paroxetine is a class D agent because of reports of an increased risk of cardiac defects
- SSRIs are potentially associated with pulmonary hypertension in newborns
    - Data are limited to studies with exposure to SSRIs after the 20th week
    - Estimated risk <1%
- SSRIs are associated with a neonatal syndrome that includes increased muscle tone, restlessness, and tremor that resolve spontaneously after several days
- TCAs are often used and are also helpful in treating insomnia; desipramine and nortriptyline are least likely to induce orthostatic hypotension

- Bupropion: mixed data; recent data have not shown risk of congenital malformations
- Mirtazapine and duloxetine: little prospective data
- Monoamine oxidase inhibitors (MAOIs): should be avoided during pregnancy because there is a risk of hypertensive crisis when combined with tocolytics

MOOD STABILIZERS

- Mood stabilizers are often continued in women with bipolar disorder during pregnancy because of the high risk of relapse
- Teratogenic risk is associated with many mood stabilizers
- Lithium: risk of Ebstein's anomaly is one in 1,000
- Valproic acid and carbamazepine: these agents should be avoided because of the risk of neural tube defects (1%–6%)
- Lamotrigine: multiple registries have collected data showing a low risk of cleft palate
- Other anticonvulsants have limited information about safety
- Reinitiation of lithium prior to delivery (after >36 weeks) has been shown to be effective for the prevention of postpartum mood episodes

ANTIPSYCHOTICS

- Typical antipsychotics: High-potency agents are recommended over low-potency agents because of an increased risk of congenital malformations with low-potency antipsychotics after the first trimester; therefore, haloperidol, perphenazine, and trifluoperazine are preferable
- Atypical Antipsychotics:
  - Little data overall
  - Olanzapine, quetiapine, risperidone, clozapine: data mostly from manufacturers and case series
  - Use of atypical antipsychotics should be limited to cases in which treatment with typical antipsychotics has not been successful

ANXIOLYTICS

- Benzodiazepines: first trimester exposure: 0.7% risk of cleft lip (10-fold risk over the general population); studies remain controversial
- Zolpidem (Ambien), zaleplon (Sonata), buspirone (BuSpar): should be avoided because of a lack of safety data

ELECTROCONVULSIVE THERAPY (ECT)

- Indicated for severe depression, affective psychosis, and catatonia in pregnancy and the postpartum period

BREASTFEEDING

- All psychotropic medications are excreted in breast milk; the concentration varies widely
- Mothers must weigh the risks of an infant's exposure to medications with benefits of breast-feeding
- Disruption in sleep from breastfeeding carries risk of relapse for women at risk for mood and psychotic disorders
- Studies of TCAs, fluoxetine, sertraline, and paroxetine have been reassuring

- Mood stabilizers: reports of neonatal toxicity with lithium, carbamazepine, and valproic acid (associated with lithium toxicity and hepatotoxicity)
- Breast-feeding very premature babies should be avoided if the mother is taking psychotropics

CONTRACEPTION

- Modafinil, carbamazepine, topiramate, and oxcarbazepine enhance oral contraceptive pills (OCPs) metabolism, rendering OCPs less effective
- Norplant metabolism is enhanced by phenobarbital
- Levels of TCAs and benzodiazepines are increased by OCPs
- Lamotrigine levels are lowered by OCPs

MENSTRUAL DISORDERS

Premenstrual Dysphoric Disorder (PMDD)

- **Definition:** A severe form of premenstrual syndrome (PMS) characterized by significant premenstrual mood disturbance causing impairment in social or occupational functioning
- **Prevalence:** 3% to 8% of women of reproductive age
- **Symptoms:** irritability, depressed mood, cravings, hot flashes
- **Differential diagnosis:** depression, anxiety, fibromyalgia, migraine, irritable bowel syndrome
- **Diagnosis:** 2 months of prospective mood charting with menstrual cycle is required for diagnosis
- **Treatment:** SSRIs during the luteal phase; also drospirenone and ethinyl estradiol (Yasmin) are approved by the Food and Drug Administration (FDA)
- **Supportive treatment:** nonsteroidal anti-inflammatory drugs (NSAIDS); reduction in caffeine, salt, sugar, nicotine, and alcohol; Ca/Mg supplements; sleep; exercise

Polycystic Ovary Syndrome (PCOS)

- **Definition:** a syndrome characterized by oligo- or amenorrhea and hyperandrogenism (hirsutism, virilization, acne)
  - Other features may include insulin resistance, obesity, hypothalamic–pituitary abnormalities, and polycystic ovaries
  - May contribute to infertility
  - Affective syndrome includes mood lability
- **Prevalence:** 10% of women
- Valproic acid has been implicated as a cause of PCOS (Joffe et al, 2006)

Geriatric Patients

- The older patient population is increasing at a rapid rate
- Decreased functional reserve affects illness presentation and course: when illness strikes, geriatric patients may quickly lose the ability to perform activities of daily living (ADLs) and to remain independent
- Be aware of multiple comorbid medical conditions and resultant drug–drug interactions

TABLE 4-5 Approach to the Evaluation of the Geriatric Patient

History and Examination
History
• Source: family members, caregivers, patient (may be less reliable); patients rarely self-present
• Presenting symptoms, psychiatric history, substance use
• Functional status: ADLs (feeding, dressing, toileting, taking medications)
• Instrumental ADLs (cooking, driving, shopping, managing finances)
• Safety at home: using stove or stairs, risk of wandering
Medical history, with special attention to:
• Falls, incontinence, gait instability, weight loss, sensory impairments
• Medical history, including vascular risk factors
• Medications: OTC medications, anticholinergics, psychiatric medications, and opiate analgesics may have mood-altering and adverse cognitive effects
Perform a through examination (medical, neurologic, full mental status examination)
Cognitive and Frontal Lobe Examinations
Cognitive functioning: orientation, attention, memory, language, executive functioning (e.g., clock-drawing, fund of knowledge)
Folstein MMSE with or without Montreal Cognitive Assessment (available at http:www.mocatest.org)
• **Abstraction:** similarities, proverbs
• **Perseveration:** go/no-go, pattern copying: cursive m's and n's, Luria motor sequence
• **Executive functioning:** attention and working memory, digit span backwards, serial sevens, spelling words backward, days of week and months backward
• **Primitive reflexes:** grasp, glabellar, suck, snout
• **Praxis:** comb hair, brush teeth, salute
• **Disinhibition and verbal fluency:** listing words starting with F in 1 minute
• Judgment of how to deal with emergency situations

ADLs, activities of daily living; MMSE, Mini-Mental State Examination; OTC, over the counter.

Psychiatric Concerns in Geriatric Patients

Cognitive Impairment

- Greatest risk factor: increasing age (especially >85 years); however, it is not a normal fact of aging
- Brief differential diagnosis: dementia, delirium, depression (cognitive impairment sometimes seen in depression, formerly called "pseudodementia"), sleep apnea

Delirium (see page 9 for more information)

- **Patients at highest risk:** age older than 65 years, brain injured (including dementia and cerebrovascular disease), postcardiac surgery, burn victims, patients withdrawing from substances, patients with autoimmune disorders
- **Common causes:** infection (especially urinary tract and pulmonary infections), constipation, hypoxia, medication effects, substances (intoxication or withdrawal), metabolic, intracerebral hemorrhage (e.g., subdural hemorrhages after a fall), sensory impairment (hearing loss, cataracts)

- **"Sundowning":** The onset or exacerbation of delirium during the evening or night with improvement or resolution during the day
- Associated with poor prognosis; symptoms may persist up to 12 months after initial hospitalization
- **Workup:** vital signs, examination, laboratory and other studies: electrolytes, urinalysis, blood culture, electrocardiographic (EKG), head computed tomography (CT) (to rule out stroke or bleed), electroencephalography (EEG)
- **Treatment:**
  - Treat the underlying cause
  - Behavioral treatment: reorient the patient (clocks, calendars on walls); use soft and low lighting at night to correct sleep–wake cycle
  - Minimize the use of restraints, but they may be necessary to prevent falls and hip fractures

TABLE 4-6 Pharmacologic Management of Acute Agitation in Geriatric Patients

Drug	Dosage	Notes
Trazodone	12.5–25.0 mg PO q6h	
Olanzapine	2.5–5.0 mg PO, IM, or SL	Avoid concurrent IM olanzapine with IM benzodiazepine
Quetiapine	12.5–25.0 mg PO	Preferable for parkinsonism
Risperidone	0.25–0.5 mg PO or liquid	
Haloperidol	0.5–1.0 mg PO or IM	
Lorazepam	0.25–0.5 mg PO or IM	

IM, intramuscular; PO, orally; SL, sublingual.

Depression

- Atypical presentation in this population:
  - More somatic symptoms (GI pain/constipation, chest pain, headache, joint pain, nausea, dizziness, fatigue or weakness), weight loss
  - Anhedonia or apathy > dysphoric mood (patients may deny being depressed)
  - Unrelenting, ruminative focus on a self-perceived cognitive impairment (despite objective evidence to the contrary) may be sign of psychotic depression
- Irritability or elevated mood may be present in patients with mood disorders and dementia
- Associated with cardiac (including after myocardial infarction [MI]) illness, neurologic illness, or cancer
- Bidirectional association with medical illness: complicates recovery from medical problems and vice versa
- Suicide after age 65 years: highest rate of any age group in the United States
- Differential diagnosis: hypothyroidism, medications (sedative–hypnotics, steroids), alcohol, dementia

- Treatment:
  - First-line antidepressants with the least drug–drug interactions: citalopram, sertraline (avoid paroxetine because of anticholinergic effects)
  - If poor sleep, weight loss, and anxiety: consider mirtazapine
  - If an urgent response is needed, especially if the patient has apathy, amotivation, and anergia, consider psychostimulants (use caution if the patient has cardiac disease)
  - Also consider venlafaxine, duloxetine, nortriptyline, and bupropion (unless the patient has high anxiety)
  - Refractory depression, psychotic depression, mania: ECT

Psychosis

- Assess for and treat any underlying delirium
- Most commonly caused by dementia and delirium followed by mood disorders (psychotic depression, mania) and chronic psychotic disorders
- Late-onset schizophrenia: onset >45 years; represents ~25% of patients with schizophrenia >65 years; associated with less severe negative symptoms; prevalence is higher in women than men; higher functioning; better cognition
- May be related to sensory impairments (visual, auditory, rarely tactile)
- AH, bizarre delusions: more commonly schizophrenia (early vs. late onset)
- VH, nonbizarre delusions: delirium, dementia
- See Below in "Special Considerations in the Treatment of Geriatric Patients" for treatment options and precautions

Other Important Geriatric Syndromes

Weight Loss

- Differential diagnosis: Failure to thrive, hypoactive delirium, apathy secondary to dementia, depression, thyroid, malignancy, dysphagia (neurologic causes, esophageal strictures)

Substance Abuse

- Alcoholism often goes unreported or overlooked; prevalence: ~10% to 20%
- Increased blood alcohol concentration relative to volume ingested because of decreased volume of distribution
- Increased risk of suicide, alcohol-related dementia, and malnutrition

Mania

- Late-life bipolar disorder: 10% develop first-onset mania after age 50 years
- Usually secondary to neurologic or other medical disease, including right temporal or frontal lesion or use of steroid medications
- Irritability or elevated mood may be present in patients with mood disorders and dementia

Anxiety Disorders

- Most common: simple phobias, panic disorder with agoraphobia, generalized anxiety disorder, OCD
- Often co-occur with depression; portend worse prognosis and a lower or delayed treatment response

Special Considerations in the Treatment of Geriatric Patients

General Principles

- Alterations in drug clearance in elderly patients increases their sensitivity to medications
- The rate of titration should start low and go slow
- Minimize polypharmacy whenever possible
- PRNs: use existing medications whenever possible to limit polypharmacy
- Resolution of symptoms requires a longer duration of treatment in geriatric patients
- Behavioral interventions and psychotherapy augment treatment response

Potential Complications of Treatment in this Population

- Increased sensitivity to side effects:
  - Sedation: limit benzodiazepines, TCAs, anticholinergics
  - Anticholinergics: avoid or limit diphenhydramine, benztropine, chlorpromazine, TCAs, thioridazine
  - Orthostasis: monitor vital signs in patients taking quetiapine, trazodone, clozapine, chlorpromazine, and TCAs
  - Extrapyramidal side effects (EPS): high doses of risperidone (>2 mg/day) have similar EPS effects as typical antipsychotic
- Benzodiazepines: use cautiously because of the potential for cognitive impairment, ataxia, fall risk, paradoxical agitation and disinhibition, and respiratory depression
- QTc prolongation is associated with many antipsychotics; check the baseline electrocardiography, replete K^+ and Mg^+
- FDA black box warning: there is an increased risk of death with typical and atypical antipsychotics for treatment of behavioral disorders in elderly patients, although they are widely used
- SSRIs are commonly associated with the syndrome of inappropriate antidiuretic hormone secretion (SIADH); also increased risk for hyponatremia with hydrochlorothiazide (HCTZ), dehydration, and the "tea and toast" diet in elderly individuals

Other Issues Specific to the Geriatric Population

- Capacity to accept treatment; decision-making ability
- Goal of care: maximize function
- Caregiver fatigue, family supports
- End-of-life issues (see page 134 for more information)
- Elder abuse (physical, sexual, psychological, financial; exploitation and neglect)
  - Patients >80 years are at highest risk
  - In 90% of cases, the abuser is a family member
  - Mandatory reporting to Adult Protective Services (APS): Elder Abuse Hotline: 800-922-2275

Medically Ill Patients

This section addresses:

- How to do a psychiatric consultation for a medical or surgical team
- The psychiatric evaluation of medically ill patients
- Psychiatric symptoms caused by medical conditions
- Psychiatric symptoms caused by medical treatment
- General principles of psychiatric treatment for medically ill patients
- Medical complications of psychiatric treatment
- See sections for evaluation and management of specific populations, including geriatrics, HIV, organ failure and transplant, cardiac illness, cancer, and neurologic illness

GUIDELINES FOR CONSULTATION ON MEDICAL AND SURGICAL WARDS

- Speak directly with the referring clinician and identify specific consult question(s)
- Review the chart and gather collateral information
- Obtain vital signs and medications lists (including PRNs and recent changes)
- Perform a thorough psychiatric evaluation, including a full mental status examination, a frontal lobe examination, and relevant physical and neurologic examinations
- Document findings and communicate directly with the primary team
- Rule out psychiatric symptoms caused by a general medical condition
- Provide psychoeducation to the patient and family and assist with aftercare
- Consider the psychological impact of medical illness and loss of functioning on the patient and family
- Make periodic follow-up visits

PSYCHIATRIC EVALUATION OF MEDICALLY ILL PATIENTS

TABLE 4-7 Approach to the Evaluation of the Medically Ill Patient

History

History of present illness:

- Sources: the patient (often poor historian), caregivers, chart, family
- Characterize the medical and psychiatric symptoms
- Onset: age, rapidity, precipitating factors (trauma, loss, medication noncompliance)
- Course: stable, progressive, deteriorating, episodic
- Determine any temporal relationship between psychiatric symptoms and medical illness
- Assess for delirium
- Assess for underlying medical causes of psychiatric symptoms
- Perform a thorough medical review of symptoms
- Determine the patient's baseline cognitive and psychiatric level of function
- Medical decision making: living will, health care proxy, DNR or DNI status, hospice eligibility

(continued)

TABLE 4-7 Approach to the Evaluation of the Medically Ill Patient (*continued*)

Medical history:
- Current and past medical problems
- Current medications and recent changes, history of adherence
- Illness course, treatment, degree and rate of loss of functioning
- History of head trauma, thyroid illness, seizures
- History of falls, syncope

Psychiatry history:
- Axis I disorders, hospitalizations, self-injurious behavior, psychotropic drug trials and response

Substance abuse history:
- Current and past use of tobacco, alcohol, illicit drugs; complications of use

General Medical and Neurologic Examination with special attention to:

Vital signs

General appearance (e.g., uncomfortable, pale, cachectic, tremulous, somnolent, pupil size): signs of recent trauma, surgical scars

Neurologic examination
- **Cranial nerves:** pupil size and reactivity, extraocular movements/nystagmus, facial symmetry, vision, hearing
- **Muscle bulk, tone, and strength:** rigidity or cogwheeling, atrophy, fasciculations, asterixis
- **Reflexes:** deep tendon reflexes, palmomental reflex, clonus
- **Coordination and gait:** Romberg, balance and retropulsion, ambulation
- **Tremor:** e.g., intention, resting, coarse

Psychiatric Mental Status Examination with special attention to:

Appearance and behavior: agitation, eye contact, calm vs. frightened
Level of arousal and orientation: alert, oriented, somnolent, stuporous, inattentive
Speech: fluent, dysarthric, rambling, rapid, incoherent
Motor activity: slowed, hyperactive, tics, tremor, weakness
Mood: angry, apathetic, depressed, fearful, tearful, irritable
Affect:, despondent, blunted, irritable, hostile
Thought process and content: linear, paranoid, loose associations, hallucinations
Judgment and insight
Cognition: orientation, concentration, confusion, short- and long-term memory
- Folstein MMSE with or without the Montreal Cognitive Assessment, clock drawing
- Frontal lobe examination: Luria maneuvers, primitive reflexes

Laboratory Studies, Imaging, and Other Diagnostic Tools

Initial basic tests: electrolytes, glucose, BUN or creatinine, liver function tests, serum and urine toxicology screens, CBC, ECG, CXR, urinalysis, HCG
Additional tests (when indicated): brain imaging, EEG, urine culture and sensitivity, vitamin B12 and folate, thyroid function tests, RPR, heavy metal screen, ANA, ESR, ammonia level, HIV testing, lumbar puncture

ANA, antinuclear antibody; BUN, blood urea nitrogen; CBC, complete blood count; CXR, chest radiography; DNR, Do Not Resuscitate; DNI, do not intubate; ECG, electrocardiography; ESR, erythrocyte sedimentation rate; HCG, human chorionic gonadotropin; HIV, human immunodeficiency virus; MMSE, Mini-Mental State Examination; RPR, rapid plasma reagin.
Adapted from Heckers S, Pasinksi RC: The patient with neuropsychiatric dysfunction. In: Stern TA, Herman JB, Slavin PL, eds. *Massachusetts General Hospital Guide to Primary Care Psychiatry*, 2nd ed. New York: McGraw-Hill; 2004:216–222.

Agitation in Medically Ill Patients

TABLE 4-8 Common Causes of Agitation in Medically Ill Patients

Disruption of basic needs:
- Hunger, thirst, pain, fear, confusion, frustration (with or without cognitive impairment), constipation
- Constipation

Delirium

Neurologic:
- Head injury
- Seizure
- Increased ICP
- Stroke
- Hemorrhage, especially if history of falls or if coagulopathic

Drugs:
- Medications: e.g., anticholinergic toxicity, benzodiazepines, steroids
- Withdrawal
- Akathisia

Infection:
- UTI, pneumonia

Vital sign instability:
- Hypertensive encephalopathy, hypotension
- Hypo- or hyperglycemia
- Hypoxia

ICP, intracranial pressure; UTI, urinary tract infection.

Treatment of Agitation

- Treat the underlying cause
- Discontinue or taper offending medications
- Symptomatic treatment: see page 13 for more information

Psychiatric Symptoms Caused by a Medical Condition

TABLE 4-9 Psychiatric Symptoms Associated with Medical Conditions

Anxiety

Cardiovascular: hypoxia, CHF, arrhythmia, mitral valve prolapse, anemia, angina
Endocrine: hypo- or hyperglycemia, hyperthyroidism, pheochromocytoma, hyperparathyroidism, Cushing's disease
Intoxication or withdrawal: caffeine, stimulants alcohol, benzodiazepines, opiates
Medications (see Table 4-10)
Metabolic: hypercalcemia, acidosis
Neurologic: seizures, vestibular dysfunction
Nutritional deficiency: niacin
Respiratory: hypoxia, COPD, pulmonary embolism

Cognitive Changes

AIDS dementia
Dementing processes
Epilepsy
Hypo- or hyperglycemia
Hyponatremia
Infection: neurosyphilis, chronic meningitis, encephalitis, prion disease
Hypo- or hyperparathyroidism
Medications (see Table 4-10)
Metabolic encephalopathies: hepatic, renal
Nutritional deficiencies
TBI or postconcussive syndrome

(continued)

TABLE 4-9 Psychiatric Symptoms Associated with Medical Conditions (*continued*)

Depression	
Catatonia **CNS process:** Parkinson's disease, Alzheimer's disease, Wilson's disease, seizure, neoplasm, poststroke depression, NPH, multiple sclerosis, infection, traumatic brain injury **Endocrine:** hypothyroidism, hyper- or hypercortisolism, hyper- or hypocalcemia **Immunologic:** SLE, RA, MS **Infectious:** lyme, syphilis, HIV/AIDS	**Intoxication, withdrawal, or chronic use** **Inflammatory illness:** IBS, fibromyalgia **Medications:** (see Table 4-10) **Metabolic:** porphyria, hepatic encephalopathy **Neoplasm:** pancreatic, paraneoplastic syndromes, frontal lobe tumors **Nutritional deficiencies:** vitamin B12, niacin, folate **Toxins:** lead, mercury
Mania	
Delirium **CNS process:** stroke, seizure, infections, neoplasm, TBI, MS, SLE **Endocrine:** hyperthyroidism, hypo- or hyperglycemia, Cushing's disease	**Infections:** Lyme disease, meningitis, HIV, neurosyphilis **Intoxication or withdrawal** **Medications:** (see Table 4-10) **Vitamin deficiencies:** vitamin B12
Psychosis	
Delirium **CNS processes:** seizure (especially temporal lobe epilepsy), neoplasm or space-occupying lesions, infection (HIV, neurosyphilis, rabies, HSV, chronic meningitis) Huntington's disease, Wilson's disease, MS, trauma, vascular malformations **Endocrine:** Cushing's disease, hyper- or hypothyroidism, hypo- or hypercalcemia	**Infections:** Lyme disease **Intoxication or withdrawal** SLE **Medications:** (see Table 4-10) **Porphyria** **Toxins:** mercury, carbon monoxide **Vitamin deficiencies:** vitamin B12

CHF, congestive heart failure; CNS, central nervous system; COPD, chronic obstructive pulmonary disease; HIV, human immunodeficiency virus; HSV, herpes simplex virus; IBS, irritable bowel syndrome; MS, multiple sclerosis; NPH, normal-pressure hydrocephalus; RA, rheumatoid arthritis; SLE, systemic lupus erythematosus; TBI, traumatic brain injury.

Psychiatric Complications of Medical Treatment

TABLE 4-10 Psychiatric Conditions Caused by Selected Medications

Anxiety

- Anticholinergic agents: benztropine, diphenhydramine
- Albuterol, bronchodilators
- α-Adrenergic antagonists
- AZT
- Bupropion
- Drug intoxication: caffeine, cannabis, cocaine, diet pills, PCP
- Drug withdrawal: alcohol, benzodiazepines, opiates
- Immunosuppressants: cyclosporine, mycophenolate (CellCept), Tacrolimus
- Interferon
- Lidocaine
- Thyroxine
- SSRIs: discontinuation or treatment initiation
- Stimulants: e.g., methylphenidate

Depression

- Antiparkinsonian: levodopa
- Barbiturates, benzodiazepines
- Cardiac: amiodarone, digitalis, diltiazem, prazosin, procainamide, beta-blockers, CCBs, reserpine, α_2-adrenergic agonists (methyldopa, clonidine)
- Chemotherapeutic agents: vincristine, vinblastine, corticosteroids, interferon, interleukin-2, asparaginase, procarbazine, tamoxifen
- Cholinergic drugs: neostigmine
- Drug abuse: chronic alcohol, sedative–hypnotics, opiates
- Drug withdrawal: cocaine, methamphetamines
- H2-blockers: ranitidine, cimetidine
- Immunosuppressants: mycophenolate (CellCept)
- Interferon
- Metoclopramide
- Oral contraceptives
- Steroids: e.g., glucocorticoids

Mania or Agitation

- Antidepressants
- AZT
- Drug intoxication
- Steroids
- Interferon
- Procainamide

Psychosis

- Anticholinergics: atropine
- Dopaminergic drugs: levodopa, ropinirole (Requip), pramipexole (Mirapex)
- Digitalis toxicity
- Drug abuse: cocaine, amphetamines, PCP, hallucinogens, anabolic steroids
- Drug withdrawal: alcohol, sedative–hypnotics
- Efavirenz
- Immunosuppressants: cyclosporine
- Interferon
- Isoniazid
- Lidocaine
- Metoclopramide
- NSAIDs
- Steroids

AZT, azidothymidine; CCB, calcium channel blocker; NSAID, nonsteroidal antiinflammatory drug; PCP, phencyclidine; SSRI, selective serotonin reuptake inhibitor.

Psychiatric Considerations in Medically Ill Patients

Depression in Medically Ill Patients

- Sadness, grief, and bereavement are normal responses to coping with illness; anhedonia, treatment refusal, social isolation, and SI are not
- **Increased morbidity and mortality:** outcomes of both depression and medical illness are negatively influenced by each other
- **Diagnosis:** use the *Diagnostic and Statistical Manual of Mental Disorders IV (DSM-IV)* criteria for major depressive disorder (MDD); because of overlap between medical illness and neurovegetative signs (anorexia, fatigue, insomnia), some advocate for using psychological symptoms (dysphoria, sadness, lack of pleasure, social isolation, refusal of treatment, SI)
- **Differential diagnosis:** fatigue, adjustment disorder, depression secondary to a general medical condition (see chart), medications (see chart)

Fatigue

- Commonly reported among medically ill patients; not a true Axis I diagnosis
- **Differential diagnosis:** anemia, untreated pain, sleep disturbance, MDD, hypothyroidism, nutritional deficits, secondary to medication use (steroids, narcotics, antiemetics, beta-blockers, radiation therapy)
- **Workup:** vital signs, complete blood count (CBC), thyroid-stimulating hormone (TSH), albumin, calcium, liver function tests (LFTs)
- **Treatment:** correct specific abnormalities; symptomatic treatment may include psychostimulants (use caution in patients with cardiovascular disease, psychosis), physical therapy, exercise, and therapy

Anxiety

- Factors distinguishing anxiety from an organic cause vs. primary anxiety: onset >35 years, lack of personal or family history, no identified stressors, poor response to anxiolytics
- **Differential diagnosis:** primary anxiety disorder, secondary to medical condition, or as a consequence of treatment (see Table 4-10)

End-of-Life Issues

KUBLER-ROSS STAGES

- Denial: the person is unwilling or unable to accept the diagnosis ("This cannot be happening to me!")
- Anger: prominent feelings of injustice ("What did I do to deserve this?")
- Bargaining: the patient begs his or her "higher power" to undo the diagnosis ("I guarantee I'll be a better person if . . .")
- Depression: the patient confronts the inevitability and reality of diagnosis and his or her helplessness to change it ("I don't even care anymore.")
- Acceptance: the patient has processed grief and can plan to move forward ("I'm ready to handle whatever comes.")

GOALS OF "END-OF-LIFE CARE"

- Issues to be addressed: treatment decisions, potential future symptoms, existential issues, concerns about the process of dying
- Include caregivers because they have similar rates of psychiatric disorders as patients with advanced disease

- Consults to consider: support groups, pain service, chaplaincy, palliative care team for symptom management and overall end-of-life concerns

Psychopharmacologic Treatment in Elderly and Medically Ill Patients

General Considerations

- Medically compromised patients have altered pharmacokinetics and pharmacodynamics
- Therefore, they may be more susceptible to adverse or life-threatening side effects
  - For example, the use of anxiolytics may cause respiratory depression
  - Medications associated with orthostatic hypotension may cause significant sequelae (e.g., falls causing hip fractures, subdural hematomas)
  - Benzodiazepines and anticholinergics may cause disinhibition and agitation
  - Many medications may worsen delirium in medically ill patients
- Medically compromised patients are also more likely to have drug–drug interactions that may cause clinically significant toxicity or underdosing (e.g., subtherapeutic antiepileptic levels)
  - Adding an inhibitor of p450 enzymes will rapidly increase the blood levels of a drug
  - Adding an inducer of p450 enzymes will lower the blood level
  - Stopping an inducer will cause an increase in blood level
  - Stopping an inhibitor will cause decrease in blood level
- Anxiolytics must be used cautiously because of the risk for respiratory depression

Guidelines for Treatment

- Review relevant conditions (e.g., ileus, cirrhosis, hypoalbuminemia, renal failure) and their effects on pharmacokinetics and pharmacodynamics of prescribed medications
- Adjust doses accordingly; consider following therapeutic levels of medications if possible
- Review possible drug–drug interactions
- Monitor for toxicity
- Start low and go slow when dosing medications but ensure therapeutic doses
- Determine which drugs are efficacious and which are unnecessary. If a drug is unnecessary, taper and discontinue it
- Remember that metabolism and clearance may fluctuate with illness course, so be vigilant for variable effects of medications

Alterations in Drug Clearance that Increase Medication Levels

- **Increased absorption:** ileus, narcotics
- **Distribution:**
  - Decreased lean body mass and total body water may lead to increased plasma concentration of water-soluble drugs

- Decreased albumin may lead to a higher percentage of unbound metabolically active drug. Diseases with low-protein states include cirrhosis, cachexia and anorexia, and nephrotic syndrome
- **Excretion**
  - Decreased hepatic enzyme activity leading to slowed metabolism causes a buildup of metabolites
  - Decreased renal function leads to a longer half-life of renally excreted drugs (lithium, gabapentin, levetiracetam)
  - See Tables 4-29 and 4-30 for chart of dose reductions in renal and hepatic failure

Alterations in Drug Clearance that Lower Drug Levels

- **Absorption:** diarrheal illness, metoclopramide, or other processes that speed gastrointestinal (GI) motility
- **Distribution:** increased total body fat leads to decreased plasma concentration and slower elimination of fat-soluble drugs

Drug–Drug Interactions

TABLE 4-11 Drug–Drug Interactions

Inducers of Metabolism	Inhibitors of Metabolism
Drugs	**Drugs**
• Barbiturates	• Antifungals (azoles)
• Carbamazepine	• Antiretrovirals
• Phenytoin	• Antimalarials
• Primidone	• Amiodarone
• Rifampin	• Beta-blockers
• Ritonavir	• CCBs
Diet and Lifestyle	• Cimetidine
• Cruciferous vegetables (e.g., cabbage, broccoli, Brussels sprouts)	• Fluoroquinolones
• Charbroiled meats	• Isoniazid
• Cigarettes	• Macrolide antibiotics
	• Quinidine
	• Phenothiazines
	• SSRIs
	• Valproic acid
	Diet
	• Grapefruit juice

CCB, calcium channel blocker; SSRI, selective serotonin reuptake inhibitor.

Specific Choices of Psychopharmacologic Treatment

GENERAL PRINCIPLE

- Medication choice is usually determined by the side effect profile, p450 interactions, and history of response

ANTIDEPRESSANTS

- Drug–drug interactions: citalopram and sertraline have the fewest drug–drug interactions; fluoxetine and fluvoxamine have the most
- Fatigue: bupropion, modafinil, stimulants can be helpful

- Anorexia, insomnia: mirtazapine can improve both
- Neuropathic pain: duloxetine or gabapentin; TCAs are helpful but are rarely used because of side effects
- Precautions:
  - SSRIs may cause decreased platelet aggregation, so use with caution in patients with hematologic impairments
  - SSRIs may cause hyponatremia, so monitor sodium, especially in patients with SIADH, risk of dehydration, or taking diuretics such as HCTZ
  - Bupropion lowers the seizure threshold; use caution in patients with brain tumors, seizure disorders, and arrhythmias
  - TCAs: can cause arrhythmias, orthostasis
  - Mirtazapine: can cause orthostasis, weight gain, and sedation

PSYCHOSTIMULANTS

- Effective for depression, opiate-induced sedation, cognitive impairment, low energy or appetite; also potentiate the analgesic effects of opiates
- Rapid onset (hours) useful in advanced illness
- Precautions: coronary artery disease, arrhythmias, seizure disorders

ANTIPSYCHOTICS

- Indications in medically ill patients with psychosis, mania, agitation, delirium, fear, anxiety, and insomnia; may be a useful adjunctive treatment for pain
- Precautions:
  - EPS and risk factors
    - Acute dystonia: male gender, age <30 years, IM administration
    - Parkinsonism: older age, female gender, Parkinson's disease
    - Akathisia: possibly advanced age and diabetes
    - Tardive dyskinesia: older age, prolonged exposure to antipsychotics, diabetes
    - Neuroleptic malignant syndrome: dehydration, agitation with or without use of restraints, IM administration, rapid discontinuation of dopamine agonists (i.e., for Parkinson's disease or restless legs syndrome)
  - Anticholinergic toxicity, orthostasis, sedation
  - QTc prolongation: monitor QTc on EKG, replete Mg and K
  - Hyponatremia, SIADH
  - Metabolic syndrome, worsening of diabetes, dyslipidemias: use with caution in patients with high body mass index (BMI), family or personal history of congestive heart disease, smoking, and hyperlipidemia
- Black box warning in elderly patients because of an increased risk of death

ANXIOLYTICS

- Consider nonbenzodiazepine anxiolytic treatment: reassurance, low-dose trazodone, gabapentin, atypical-antipsychotics
- Benzodiazepines: effective for short-term treatment of anxiety, agitation, withdrawal; use benzodiazepines with shorter half-lives in the medical setting
- Precautions:
  - Agitation and disinhibition in patients with brain damage (including geriatric patients)
  - Sedation: monitor for additive effects with opiates, other sedating drugs, and altered metabolism; monitor respiratory rate

- Respiratory depression: monitor respiration, oxygen saturation
- Dependence: patients with prolonged hospital courses may become physiologically dependent; be vigilant for withdrawal

MEDICAL COMPLICATIONS OF PSYCHIATRIC TREATMENT

Life-Threatening Complications of Psychiatric Treatment

- Neuroleptic malignant syndrome
- Serotonin syndrome
- Lithium overdose
- TCA overdose
- Benzodiazepine withdrawal
- Hyponatremia
- Torsades des pointes
- Hepatitis
- Seizure
- Agranulocytosis
- Stevens-Johnson syndrome
- Tyramine crisis (from MAOI)

Common Medical Complications of Psychiatric Treatment by System

ANTICHOLINERGIC EFFECTS

- Tachycardia, constipation, dry mouth (delirium at toxic doses)
- Common in TCAs and some SSRIs such as paroxetine (none in fluoxetine), low-potency antipsychotics, olanzapine, benztropine, mirtazapine

CARDIOVASCULAR

- Arrhythmia
  - TCAs are structurally similar to class I antiarrhythmics; they increase PR, QRS, and QTc. Use with caution in patients with ventricular arrhythmias
  - TCAs may be lethal in overdose (look for QRS widening on EKG)
  - Lithium may cause first-degree atrioventricular (AV) block and flatted or inverted T waves on EKG
  - QTc prolongation may be seen with haloperidol, low-potency antipsychotics, TCAs, and other antipsychotics at high doses (ziprasidone, risperidone)
  - Psychostimulants may cause arrhythmia or hypertension
- Hypertension
  - Venlafaxine, stimulants, and bupropion may be associated with hypertension
  - Hypertensive crisis may be seen with MAOIs, tyramine, and stimulants
- Orthostasis
  - TCAs, MAOIs, quetiapine, trazodone, mirtazapine, low-potency antipsychotics (e.g., chlorpromazine, clozapine)
- Myocarditis or cardiomyopathy
  - Clozapine: rare but serious (0.7%–1.2% incidence)

DERMATOLOGIC

- Stevens-Johnson syndrome: lamotrigine, carbamazepine, valproic acid
- Photosensitivity: most psychotropics
- Acne: lithium
- Sweating: SSRIs and SNRIs

ENDOCRINOLOGIC

- Weight gain: atypical antipsychotics may cause metabolic syndrome

- Glucose intolerance: antipsychotics, valproic acid; rare spontaneous diabetic ketoacidosis (DKA) with atypical antipsychotics
- Thyroid dysfunction: lithium
- Hyperprolactinemia: atypical antipsychotics, especially risperidone

GASTROINTESTINAL

- Nausea is common with many medications
- Pancreatitis: rare with valproic acid, clozapine, olanzapine, risperidone
- Hepatotoxicity: valproic acid, anticonvulsants, nefazodone, Kava root
- Hyperammonemia or hepatic encephalopathy: valproic acid
- Sialorrhea: clozapine, low-potency antipsychotics (associated with aspiration pneumonia)

HEMATOLOGIC

- Small bleeding risk from the antiplatelet effects of SSRIs, gingko, and ginger root
- Agranulocytosis: clozapine, valproic acid

METABOLIC

- Hyponatremia or SIADH: carbamazepine and oxcarbazepine are common causes (prevalence ≤29%); SSRIs (especially in combination with thiazides, dehydration)
- Dyslipidemia: antipsychotics

RENAL

- Nephrotoxicity: lithium (worsened with NSAIDs, angiotensin-converting enzyme inhibitors, thiazide diuretics)
- Nephrogenic diabetes insipidus: lithium

REPRODUCTIVE AND SEXUAL

- See Chapter 5 for more information about for teratogenic drugs
- Priapism: trazodone
- Sexual dysfunction: antidepressants
- PCOS: proposed link with valproic acid
- Reduced efficacy of OCPs: St. John's Wort, modafinil, carbamazepine, topiramate, oxcarbazepine

RESPIRATORY

- Respiratory depression: benzodiazepines; additive effects with TCAs, sedating antipsychotics, alcohol

Cancer

Approximately 50% of patients with advanced cancer meet the criteria for a psychiatric disorder.

Depression and Cancer

Depression

- The rate of MDD among inpatients with cancer is approximately 25%
- The rates of MDD are highest among patients with pancreatic, lung, head and neck, and liver cancer and in those with leukemia.

(continued)

TABLE 4-12 Considerations with History Taking in Cancer Patients

Cancer Illness and Course	
• When and how the cancer diagnosis was made • Current cancer stage (active vs. remission, type and stage) • Risk factors for cancer type (alcohol, tobacco) • Cancer treatment: chemotherapy, radiation, involvement of brain or CSF, history of lumbar puncture, bone marrow transplant	• Coping • Fatigue, pain • Delirium, depression, anxiety, mania, and psychosis • Complications of cancer or treatment: fatigue, nausea, vomiting, diarrhea, neutropenia (with infections or fever)

CSF, cerebrospinal fluid.

(continued)

Rates increase with tumor burden and disease within the brain or cerebrospinal fluid (CSF)

- Other risk factors: poor social supports, history of substance abuse, history of other psychiatric or medical illnesses
- Untreated depression is associated with decreased quality of life, decreased compliance, and increased morbidity and mortality
- Chemotherapeutic agents associated with depressed mood: vincristine, vinblastine, corticosteroids, interferon, interleukin-2, asparaginase, procarbazine, tamoxifen
- **Differential diagnosis:** chronic or acute pain, fatigue, metabolic disturbances, delirium, medications, tumor advancement to the brain or CSF. Adjustment disorder is the most common Axis I diagnosis among cancer patients
- **Workup:** TSH, cortisol, calcium, ionized calcium, vitamin B12, folate, neuroimaging, lumbar puncture
- **Treatment:** rule out and treat organic cause; consider psychotherapy, support groups, and medication (see Treatment section below)

DELIRIUM AND CANCER

See page 9 for general information about delirium.

TABLE 4-13 Selected Causes of Delirium in Cancer Patients

Brain tumors:
- Metastases: lung, melanoma, renal, breast, colorectal, thyroid, testicular cancer; more common than primary lesions

Leptomeningeal disease:
- Associated with melanoma, breast, and lung cancers

Medications:
- Steroids, immunosuppressant drugs (cyclosporine, tacrolimus, amphotericin B), benzodiazepines, opiates

Metabolic:
- Hypocalcemia: associated with bone metastases, ectopic PTHrP
- Hyponatremia: associated with SIADH; seen in small cell lung cancer, mesothelioma, pancreatic cancer, lymphoma, leukemia, infections, brain tumors, medications (SSRIs, carbamazepine, TCAs, phenothiazines)

(continued)

TABLE 4-13 Selected Causes of Delirium in Cancer Patients (*continued*)
Paraneoplastic disorders
Seizure
Stem cell transplant: • Metabolic abnormalities, infectious causes, engraftment syndrome • Immunosuppressant drugs
Toxic leukoencephalopathy: • White matter injury caused by cancer treatment; frontal lobes most affected, seen on T2-weighted MRI • Most commonly associated with methotrexate, carmustine, cisplatin, fludarabine, ifosfamide, cytarabine, fluorouracil

MRI, magnetic resonance imaging; PTHrP, parathyroid hormone–related protein; SIADH, syndrome of inappropriate antidiuretic hormone secretion; SSRI, selective serotonin reuptake inhibitor; TCA, tricyclic antidepressant.

Neuropsychiatric Effects of Cancer Treatments

TABLE 4-14 Neuropsychiatric Effects of Cancer Treatments	
Cytokines	
Interferon-α	• May lead to depression, hypomania, cognitive impairment, fatigue or sickness syndrome, and psychosis • Side effects are responsive to psychotropic agents • May inhibit metabolism of p450 enzymes CYP1A2, CYP2C19, CYP2D6 • Check TSH level because the agent may be associated with autoimmune thyroiditis
Interleukin-2	• Delirium, flu-like side effects, hypothyroidism • Neurotoxicity is dose dependant
Chemotherapy	
5-Flurouracil	• Fatigue is the most common side effect; may also lead to cerebellar dysfunction and encephalopathy • If toxic, give high-dose IV thymidine
Androgen blockade (Leuprolide, Goserelin, Flutamide)	• Hot flashes, fatigue, mood disturbances
Anti-estrogens (Tamoxifen, Toremifene, Anastrozole, Letrozole, Exemestane)	• Hot flashes, insomnia, mood changes; at high doses, may cause confusion
Asparaginase	• Depression, lethargy, delirium
Carmustine	• May cause delirium at high doses
Carboplatin	• Neurotoxicity only at high doses

(continued)

TABLE 4-14 Neuropsychiatric Effects of Cancer Treatments (*continued*)

Chemotherapy	
Cisplatin	• Reversible posterior leukoencephalopathy; toxicity is associated with cortical blindness
Cytarabine	• High-dose IV treatment may lead to confusion, obtundation, seizures, coma, cerebellar dysfunction, and leukoencephalopathy, especially in those who are elderly or with renal impairment
Gemcitabine	• Fatigue
Glucocorticoids	• Insomnia, depression, mania, psychosis, irritability
Ifosfamide	• Transient delirium, seizures, cerebellar signs that improve within days after treatment with thiamine or methylene blue; patients with kidney or liver impairment at higher risk
Kinase signaling enzyme inhibitors (Imatinib, Bevacizumab, Thalidomide)	• Confusion, fatigue, papilledema • Reversible posterior leukoencephalopathy • Drowsiness or somnolence is dose related, decreased libido, confusion
Methotrexate	• Associated with neurotoxicity when administered intrathecally or via a high-dose IV route; usually reversible and related to duration and peak level; higher rates in those with history of cranial radiation and leptomeningeal disease • Folinic acid (leucovorin) is antidote
Paclitaxel	• Seizures and transient encephalopathy • Used in conjunction with steroids
Procarbazine	• A weak MAOI • When starting an antidepressant, must consider timing of procarbazine or serious interaction may occur • Disulfiram-like effect: avoid alcohol
Vincristine, Vinblastine, Vinorelbine	• Neurotoxicity is dose related and reversible; fatigue and malaise are common

IV, intravenous; MAOI, monoamine oxidase inhibitor; TSH, thyroid-stimulating hormone.

Psychopharmacologic Considerations in Cancer Patients

See page 131 for general guidelines on treatment.

Specific Considerations in Cancer Patients:

- SSRIs may cause decreased platelet aggregation; use caution with hematologic disease (e.g., during chemotherapy)

- SSRIs may cause hyponatremia; monitor sodium in patients with brain and small cell lung cancer
- Bupropion lowers the seizure threshold; use caution in patients with central nervous system (CNS) involvement
- Use of valproate may lead to agranulocytosis and thrombocytopenia (avoid in patients undergoing chemotherapy)

Selected Drug Interactions in Cancer Patients

- Carbamazepine, phenytoin, and phenobarbital may all induce p450 enzymes, leading to decreased levels of antineoplastic taxanes, vinca alkaloids, methotrexate, teniposide, camptothecin, narcotics, antidepressants, antipsychotics, and antibiotics
- Valproate increases the toxicity of etoposide and the nitrosoureas
- Cisplatin and corticosteroids decrease phenytoin levels
- Methotrexate decreases valproate levels
- 5-Flurouracil increases phenytoin levels

Cardiac Illness

- Anxiety and depression are associated with cardiac morbidity and mortality
- Depression is associated with the onset of coronary artery disease (CAD) in previously healthy individuals and with the progression of CAD in patients with stable cardiac disease
- Depression after an MI or cardiac surgery is associated with an increased risk in mortality and adverse cardiovascular events

TABLE 4-15 Considerations with History Taking in Cardiac Patients

Cardiac Illness and Course
• Onset, course, and cause: MI, CHF, AF • Cardiac events, including history of intubation, resuscitation, cardioversion • Procedures, including IABP, defibrillator, pacemaker, or stents (bare metal vs. drug eluting); AICD discharges
Medical History and Medications
• Fatigue, exercise intolerance, dyspnea, diaphoresis, palpitations, PND, orthopnea, claudication, peripheral edema, RUQ discomfort, insomnia, falls, disequilibrium, confusion, anorexia • Comorbidities: diabetes, hypertension, dyslipidemia, peripheral vascular disease, stroke • Anticoagulation: aspirin, warfarin, clopidogrel

AF, atrial fibrillation; AICD, automated implantable cardioverter defibrillator; CHF, congestive heart failure; IABP, intraaortic balloon pump; MI, myocardial infarction; PND, paroxysmal nocturnal dyspnea; RUQ, right upper quadrant.

Psychiatric Concerns in Cardiac Patients

TABLE 4-16 Psychiatric Sequelae of Cardiac Illness

Cardiac Illness	Psychiatric Manifestations
CAD	MDD, anxiety (including panic disorder and generalized anxiety disorder)
Atrial and ventricular arrhythmias	Anxiety, panic disorder
Post-MI	MDD, anxiety, PTSD
CHF	MDD, anxiety
Cardiac surgery (CABG, valve replacement)	MDD, anxiety, delirium, PTSD
AICD	Anxiety (increased anxiety with increased incidence of discharges), PTSD symptoms, depressive symptoms
Pacemakers	Anxiety, depressive symptoms
IABP	Delirium, anxiety
LVAD	MDD, delirium

AICD, automatic implanted cardiac defibrillator; CABG, coronary artery bypass grafting; CAD, coronary artery disease; CHF, congestive heart failure; IABP, intraaortic balloon pump; LVAD, left ventricular assist devices; MDD, major depressive disorder; MI, myocardial infarction; PTSD, posttraumatic stress disorder.

Psychiatric Illnesses Associated with Cardiac Illness

Anxiety

- Anxiety has been correlated with cardiac morbidity and mortality
  - Anxiety → increased catecholamine levels → elevated vital signs → harmful cardiovascular effects
  - Anxiety → decreased heart rate variability → increased risk of arrhythmia

Treatment of Anxiety in Patients with Cardiac Illness

- Maintain a low threshold for treating anxiety in cardiac patients
- Rule out a medical cause of anxiety (e.g., arrhythmia, hypoxia, withdrawal)
- See page 52 for treatment of anxiety. Avoid benzodiazepines in patients with delirium, dementia, and traumatic brain injury

Depression in Cardiac Patients

- Depressive symptoms may predict cardiac morbidity and mortality in cardiac patients
- **An atypical presentation** common after MI depression: hostility, listlessness, withdrawal
- **Risk factors:** smoking, hypertension, female gender, social isolation, medical complications during acute hospitalization, history of depression

Proposed Mechanism for Link Between Depressive Symptoms and Cardiac Morbidity

- Depression may lead to physiologic sequelae (inflammation, increased platelet activity, hypothalamic–pituitary–adrenal axis dysfunction, elevated catecholamines, abnormal heart rate variability) and behavioral sequelae (high-fat diet, continued smoking, sedentary lifestyle, medication nonadherence, reduced rehabilitation attendance), further leading to cardiac morbidity and mortality

Principles of Treatment for Depression in Cardiac Patients

- For patients with onset of depressive symptoms after MI or cardiac surgery, have the patient follow up in 2 to 3 weeks, reevaluate, and consider pharmacologic intervention at that time
- Indications for earlier prescription of antidepressants: depression with SI, depression that interferes with rehabilitation or self-care, history of severe depression, onset of depression that preceded admission for a total of 2 weeks or more
- SSRIs are effective and have been shown to have the safest cardiac profile
- A substudy of the Sertraline AntiDepressant Heart Attack Trial (SADHAT) showed reductions in platelet or endothelial activation in patients treated with sertraline, suggesting an additional benefit of SSRIs in ischemic heart disease via reduction in platelet aggregation

Delirium in Cardiac Patients

TABLE 4-17 Selected Causes of Delirium in Cardiac Patients

Central Nervous System Hypoperfusion	Medications
• Acute MI or ischemia • CVA • Hypovolemia • Hypoxia • Relative hypotension • IABP • LVAD	• Digoxin toxicity • Narcotic analgesics • Benzodiazepines • Anticholinergic medications • H2 blockers • Anesthetics and sedatives (ICU patients)
Other General Medical Conditions	**Illicit Substances or Withdrawal**
• Electrolyte abnormalities • Hypertensive encephalopathy • Infections, stroke, seizure	

CVA, cerebrovascular accident; IABP, intraaortic balloon pump; ICU, intensive care unit; LVAD, left ventricular assist devices; MI, myocardial infarction.

Adapted from Huffman JC, Stern TA, Januzzi JL: The psychiatric management of patients with cardiac disease. In: Stern TA, Fricchione GL, Cassem NH, et al, eds. *Massachusetts General Handbook of General Hospital Psychiatry.* Philadelphia: Mosby; 2004:556.

Pharmacologic Treatment of Delirium in Cardiac Patients

- See page 9 for general treatment principles
- **First-line treatment:** intravenous (IV) haloperidol is the drug of choice in agitated, paranoid, or hyperactive patients with delirium

- Check the QTc interval before initiation
  - Haloperidol may cause QTc prolongation, increasing the risk of torsades de pointes
  - If the QTc >500, consider alternative treatment
- Check potassium and magnesium levels and correct if necessary
- The initial dose of haloperidol should be between 0.5 and 10 mg based on the patient's level of agitation, size, and age
  - Double the dose every 30 minutes until the patient is calm
  - After the effective dose is determined, use it for future episodes
- **Second-line treatment:** sublingual olanzapine or risperidone wafers; if the patient is willing to take oral medications, olanzapine, risperidone, or quetiapine may be used
- **Third-line treatment:** if the risks of antipsychotic use outweigh the benefits (e.g., because of a prolonged QTc) and the patient requires immediate sedation, narcotics and benzodiazepines may be used temporarily. Use of standing or oral valproate may also be an option in the treatment of agitation and delirium in this setting

NEUROPSYCHIATRIC EFFECTS OF TREATMENTS FOR CARDIAC ILLNESS

TABLE 4-18 Psychiatric Side Effects of Cardiovascular Medications*

Medication	Side Effects
Beta-blockers	Fatigue, lethargy, decreased libido, insomnia; minimal association with depression
α-Adrenergic agonists (clonidine)	Fatigue, sedation
α_1-Adrenergic antagonists	Fatigue, depression, sleep disturbance, anxiety
CCBs	Fatigue
Nitrates	None
Thiazide diuretics	Fatigue, weakness, delirium and psychosis (secondary to hyponatremia and hypocalcemia)
Furosemide (long-term use)	Wernicke's encephalopathy (secondary to thiamine deficiency)
Carbonic anhydrase inhibitor (acetazolamide)	Fatigue and delirium (in patients with renal failure)
Amiodarone	Fatigue and depression (via thyroid effects)
Steroids	Depression, mania, psychosis, delirium
ACE inhibitors	Mania, psychosis, delirium
Clopidogrel	Fatigue
Coumadin	Fatigue, lethargy, interactions with Ψ medications
Procainamide	Fatigue, delirium, mania
Quinidine	Delirium secondary to cinchonism
Digitalis	Visual hallucinations (yellow rings around objects), depression, delirium
Lidocaine	Delirium, anxiety, confusion, psychotic symptoms
Methyldopa	Fatigue, sedation, weak association with depression
Reserpine	Fatigue, sedation, weak association with depression
Angiotensin II receptor blockers	None

ACE, angiotensin-converting enzyme; CCB, calcium channel blocker. Adapted from Huffman JC, Stern TA: Neuropsychiatric consequences of cardiovascular medications. *Dialogues Clin Neurosci* 2007;9:57–73.

HIV/AIDS Psychiatry

- **Epidemiology:** ~1.1 million people were living with HIV in the United States in 2007
- Psychiatric and substance use disorders are common comorbidities of HIV infection, complicating both diagnosis and treatment
- Many neurologic manifestations of HIV are AIDS-defining illnesses
- Psychiatrists are frequently called for behavioral problems, delirium, psychosis, or assistance with coping

HIV Treatment with Highly Active Antiretroviral Treatment (HAART)

- Triple therapy: two nucleoside reverse transcriptase inhibitors (NRTIs) plus either a protease inhibitor (PI) or a non-nucleoside reverse transcriptase inhibitor (NNRTI)
- Goal of treatment: preserve cellular immunity (CD4 count >350) and control viral replication (viral load nondetectable)
- Department of Health and Human Services guidelines for first-line HAART are updated regularly and are available at http://www.aidsinfo.nih.gov

The current antiretroviral drug list is available from http://www.fda.gov/oashi/aids/virals.html.

TABLE 4-19 Considerations with History Taking in Patients with HIV

HIV Illness and Course
• Transmission category: how infected? • When diagnosed? Initial presentation and CD4 nadir? Which HIV cohort (recently infected or long-term survivor)? • Common medical comorbidities: HIV or HAART-induced sensory neuropathy; HIV with HCV coinfection; fatigue • History of opportunistic infections • Coping: cognitive style, personality style, experience of stigma, HIV impact (disability, medical illness burden), suicidality • Premorbid cognitive function with or without decline
Medical History and Medications
• Current HIV treatment: HAART regimen (off, new, stable), prophylactic medications; current HIV control (CD4/viral load); medication adherence and barriers (psychiatric illness, financial, active drug use) • Risk factors for metabolic syndrome
Social History
• Past and current sexual history: monogamous, status of partner, condoms, drug use before and during sexual activity; sex for drugs or money • Substance abuse

HAART, highly active antiretroviral therapy; HCV, hepatitis C virus; HIV, human immunodeficiency virus.

Neuropsychiatric Manifestations of HIV/AIDS

TABLE 4-20 Neuropsychiatric Manifestations of HIV/AIDS

Neurologic Complication	Etiology (CD4 Count)	Symptoms
Space-occupying lesions	*Toxoplasmosis* (<200), CNS lymphoma (<50–100), progressive multifocal leukoencephalopathy (<50–100)	Focal deficits, headache, delirium
Meningitis or encephalitis	CMV (<50–100), *Cryptococcus* (<200), bacterial (including *Listeria*), viral (HSV, <500), TB, lymphomatous	Fever, headache, stiff neck, photophobia, lethargy, delirium, motor sensory deficits
Neurosyphilis	*Treponema pallidum*	Meningitis, cranial nerve palsies, visual changes, seizures, dementia, tabes dorsalis

CNS, central nervous system; HSV, herpes simplex virus; TB, tuberculosis; CMV, cytomegalovirus

HIV/AIDS–Associated Mania

- **Definition:** Clinical mania with cognitive impairment in late-stage AIDS with no personal or family history of bipolar disorder
  - Accompanied by significant psychosis, mood often irritable > euphoria, sleep disturbance, and confusion
  - Must rule out delirium (see page 9 for more information)
- **Treatment:** HAART and mood-stabilizing antipsychotic

HIV-Associated Dementia Complex (HADC)

- Subcortical dementia characterized by mood, memory and motor symptoms, CD4 nadir <200
- Mood: apathy, depression, anxiety, hypomania, disinhibition, poor judgment, change in personality
- Memory: impaired memory, concentration, and attention
- Motor: mental and psychomotor slowing, incoordination, gait disturbance
- Treatment: viral suppression, symptom management

Minor Cognitive Motor Disorder (MCMD)

- Milder symptoms than HADC, word-finding difficulties, forgetfulness, less sharp, less efficient
- Treatment: viral suppression

Neuropsychiatric Side Effects of HAART and Other HIV Medications

HAART

- Most HAART medications cause headaches, insomnia, and fatigue
- Common (50%) side effects of efavirenz: headache, insomnia, somnolence, depression, abnormal or vivid dreams, hallucinations, impaired concentration
  - Serious side effects: agitation, persecutory delusions, mania, aggressive behavior, SI, suicide attempts, seizure (rare)

- Higher prevalence of side effects with very high plasma level (20% of African Americans have the CYP2B6 allele, resulting in increased efavirenz levels
- Azidothymidine (AZT): anxiety, confusion, mania
- D-drugs (d4T, ddI, ddC): pain (secondary to peripheral neuropathy)
- Isoniazid: psychosis (prevent with vitamin B6)

CONSIDERATIONS IN PRESCRIBING PSYCHIATRIC MEDICATIONS

General Guidelines

- See page 131 for general principles
- Review medication list and identify major inducers and inhibitors of metabolism
  - HAART: all PIs inhibit metabolism of psychotropics; efavirenz induces metabolism of psychotropics
  - Antibiotics: many azole and macrolide antibiotics are strong 3A4 inhibitors
  - Rifamycins (for tuberculosis or mycobacterium avium complex) are pan inducers
- Use psychotropic plasma levels if concerned about drug interactions
- Review over-the-counter and herbal preparations

Specific Medication Considerations

- Second-generation antipsychotics: overlapping metabolic toxicity with HAART, so follow weight, lipids, and glucose and avoid quetiapine for insomnia
- Clozapine: monitor for added bone marrow toxicity and metabolic syndrome
- Lithium: use caution in patients with advanced AIDS because of an increased risk of toxicity (and higher sensitivity to even normal blood levels)
- Valproic acid: consider concomitant liver toxicity of PIs; hepatitis C coinfection may increase AZT levels
- Carbamazepine: discuss with the patient's HIV doctor before use because of pan induction of P450 and toxic epidermal necrolysis (TEN); consider oxcarbazepine
- An efavirenz-based regimen may induce methadone metabolism, precipitating opiate withdrawal

Neurologic Illness

- Patients with neurologic illnesses often have overlapping psychiatric symptoms
- Suspect neurologic lesion (or other organic illness) with acute or subacute onset of psychiatric symptoms in adults
- Pharmacologic treatment should done with caution because of an increased sensitivity to medication changes and paradoxical agitation or disinhibition
- Drug–drug interactions are common with many anticonvulsants
- This section addresses the psychiatric symptoms and treatment of:
  - Stroke
  - Traumatic brain injury
  - Movement disorders (Parkinson's disease and Huntington's disease)
  - Multiple sclerosis
  - Epilepsy

TABLE 4-21 Additional History in a Patient with Neurologic Illness

Neurologic Illness and Course

- History of symptoms: onset, course, and cause (e.g., trauma, stroke)
- Determine baseline cognitive function
- Assess for changes in mood, personality, cognition, and memory
- Assess for symptoms of a mood, anxiety, or psychotic disorder
- Degree of functional impairments (gait, self-care)
- History of falls, orthostasis, headache, sensory impairments (gait, hearing, vision, dysphagia), vascular risk factors
- History of seizures, head trauma, migraines

TABLE 4-22 Neurologic Conditions that Mimic Psychiatric Symptoms

Condition	Characteristics	Associated Lesion
Expressive aprosodias	• Monotonous speech • Patient may appear withdrawn or depressed	Right frontal lobe
Abulia	• Loss of will or determination	Frontal lobes and basal ganglia
Pseudobulbar affect	• Frequent laughing or crying spells (emotional incontinence), often inappropriate to context • Associated with pseudobulbar palsy: dysphasia, dysarthria, facial weakness	Corticobulbar tract injury Associated with multiple sclerosis, ALS, brain injury
Catastrophic reactions	• Severe desperation and frustration • High correlation with poststroke depression (~75% are co-occurring)	Anterior subcortical and left cortical structures
Anosognosia	• Lack of awareness or denial of deficit	Right parietal lobe
Aphasia	• Loss of ability to produce or comprehend language • Patient may appear withdrawn, irritable	Lesions of dominant hemisphere; Broca's and Wernicke's
Palinopsia	• Recurrent images in left visual field of objects, scenes, or people • "Visual echoes"	Right-sided occipital and parietal lesions
Peduncular hallucinations	• Visual hallucinations • Also associated with sedation and oculomotor palsies • Typically nonfrightening images (e.g., children)	Pontine and midbrain lesions involving the cerebral peduncles
Charles Bonnet syndrome	• Hallucinations of benign, familiar objects, usually in elderly patients with visual loss	Multifactorial chronic visual loss
Micropsia or macropsia	• Perception that objects are smaller or bigger than in reality	Temporal lobes, occipital lobe, visual association cortex lesions (temporoparietal junction)

ALS, amyotrophic lateral sclerosis.

TABLE 4-23 Common Neurologic Causes of Visual Hallucinations

• Blindness (including palinopsia, Anton's syndrome) • Delirium tremens • Delirium • Dementia (Lewy Body > Parkinson's disease > Alzheimer's disease) • Hypnopompic (awakening) and hypnagogic (falling asleep) hallucinations	• Illusions: increased risk with visual impairment • Medicines: L-Dopa, digoxin • Migraine with aura • Peduncular hallucinosis • Seizures (frontal, complex partial, occipital)

Adapted from Kaufman D: *Clinical Neurology for Psychiatrists.* Philadelphia: WB Saunders; 2001:291.

TABLE 4-24 Brain Regions Associated with Patterns of Behavioral Abnormalities

Frontal	Language: motor aphasia (L), confabulation Affect: apathy, inappropriate behavior, disinhibition, motor aprosodia (R), irritability, abulia Memory: working memory Executive: attention, planning Motor: paresis, abulia, echopraxia, perseveration, release signs
Parietal	Language: dyslexia (L), dysgraphia (L) Affect: sensory aprosodia (R) Memory: impaired attention (R), dyscalculia (L) Motor: dyspraxia (R) Other: prosopagnosia, hemineglect (R)
Temporal	Language: sensory aphasia (L) Memory: impaired encoding or recall of information Affect: mood changes, anxiety/fear Other: hallucinations, prosopagnosia (L, R), finger agnosia (L)
Occipital	Visual hallucinations Anton's syndrome (cortical blindness with neglect of visual loss)
Striatum	Language: dysarthria, caudate nucleus (L): fluent aphasia Motor: extrapyramidal movement disorder
Thalamus	Language: confabulation; anterolateral thalamus: logorrheic aphasia Memory: impaired encoding or recall of information, impaired attention

L, left; R, right.

Adapted from Huffman J, Smith FA, Stern TA: Patients with neurologic conditions: seizure, cerebrovascular disease, and traumatic brain injury. In: Stern TA, Fricchione GL, Cassem NH, et al, eds. *Massachusetts General Hospital Handbook of General Hospital Psychiatry*, 5th ed. Philadelphia: Mosby; 2004:466.

POSTSTROKE DEPRESSION AND OTHER AXIS I DISORDERS

Poststroke Depression (PSD)

- Diagnosis follows standard *DSM-IV* criteria for major depression
- Historically associated with left frontal cortex and left basal ganglia lesions; newer data do not support this

- About 20% of poststroke patients meet criteria for MDD, and 20% meet criteria for minor depression
- Risk factors for PSD: history of depression, premorbid impairment, living alone, poststroke social isolation, and (possibly) female gender
- Comorbid depression has been shown to have a negative impact on functional recovery
- **Treatment:**
  - Multidisciplinary: combinations of physical therapy, occupational therapy, speech therapy, and cognitive rehabilitation with or without psychopharm-aceuticals, psychostimulants, or ECT
  - SSRIs and psychostimulants are first-line treatments
  - TCAs are also effective but should be used with caution because of anticholinergic effects

Other Poststroke Psychiatric Disorders

- Mania: rare: (<1% of stroke patients); may be associated with a right orbitofrontal lesion
- Anxiety: common; ~25% poststroke patients; often coexists with PSD
  - Psychosis: uncommon (1%–2% of poststroke patients); may be associated with right temporoparietal lesions; often associated with seizures

TRAUMATIC BRAIN INJURY (TBI)

- Neuropsychiatric sequelae: cognitive impairment, personality changes, Axis I disorders
- Risk factors for neuropsychologic symptoms: severity of injury, history of TBI, older age, lower IQ, comorbid substance abuse

EPIDEMIOLOGY OF TBI

- Major cause of death and disability in the United States; 1.6 million head injuries per year
- Motor vehicle collisions cause 45% of TBI cases (increased risk with young men and with alcohol)
- US veterans returning from Iraq and Afghanistan: ~18% have TBI; also highly associated with PTSD and depression

Postconcussion Syndrome (PCS)

- **Definition:** common syndrome presenting with headache, dizziness, cognitive impairment, and neuropsychiatric symptoms
- Neuropsychiatric symptoms: anxiety, fatigue, depression, intolerance to noise, irritability, impaired concentration and memory, and sleep disorders
- The risk of PCS does not correlate with the severity of the injury
- Approximately 15% to 20% patients meet criteria for psychiatric disease (depression, anxiety, or PTSD)
- Clinical diagnosis is made by exclusion; neuroimaging results are typically negative
- Analgesia overuse and rebound headaches are common

Personality Changes or "Frontal Lobe Syndrome"

- **Prevalence:** ~23% of adult patients with TBI
- **Symptoms:** labile affect, disinhibition, poor social judgment, apathy, lewd behavior, loss of social graces, perseveration, aggressive behavior, paranoia, inattention to personal hygiene

- Causes significant clinical, occupational, or social distress
- Patients often have little insight into these changes; involving family members facilitates diagnosis and treatment and allows for support of the caregivers

Axis I Disorders in Traumatic Brain Injury

- Associated with worse outcomes across domains, so early diagnosis and treatment is key
- Cognitive and behavioral deficits may mimic mood or psychotic symptoms, so neuropsychological assessment and careful diagnosis are important

Depression

- **Prevalence:** 12% to 44% of TBI patients
- **Symptoms:** fatigue, distractibility, anger, irritability, rumination
- Increased risk of suicide;15% of patients make an attempt in the first 5 years
- Comorbid with TBI-related anxiety disorders (11%)

Mania and Psychosis

- Mania: may be associated with right temporal and orbitofrontal lesions
- Psychosis: associated with frontal and temporal injuries
- There is a 3% to 9% incidence of post-TBI psychosis in acute period or after 1 to 2 years (data are controversial)
- Rule out seizure, delirium, steroid-induced psychosis or mania

Treatment of TBI

- Use a multidisciplinary approach. including behavioral treatment with or without pharmacology for specific symptom reduction
- "Start low and go slow." (TBI patients are often highly sensitive to medications.)
- Depression and anxiety: SSRIs are well tolerated
- Headache in PCS: amitriptyline is the treatment of choice
- Mood stabilization: anticonvulsants (e.g., valproic acid and carbamazepine) are preferred to lithium (because of increased side effects with lithium)
- Avoid medications that lower the seizure threshold (e.g., bupropion)
- Use with caution:
  - Medications that are highly sedating, anticholinergic, or cause significant orthostasis (e.g., TCAs, barbiturates, clozapine)
  - Benzodiazepines and barbiturates may cause paradoxical agitation and disinhibition
  - Psychostimulants: useful for depression and concentration impairments but may precipitate agitation, paranoia, paradoxical dysphoria
  - Lithium: associated with increased toxic side effects

PARKINSON'S DISEASE (PD)

- **Definition:** a chronic, progressive neurodegenerative disorder that presents with resting tremor, rigidity, brady- or akinesia, and gait disturbance
- **Prevalence:** 2.5% of the geriatric population

- **Differential diagnosis:** parkinsonism (secondary to medication, brain injury, or toxins) dementias, prion disease, alcoholic cerebellar degeneration
- **Pathophysiology:** degeneration of dopaminergic neurons in the substantia nigra
- **Treatment:** increase dopaminergic tone via:
  - Levodopa (with inhibitors of its metabolism, e.g., carbidopa or entacapone)
  - Dopamine agonists (e.g., bromocriptine)
  - Inhibitors of the metabolism of dopamine (e.g., selegiline)

Depression in Parkinson's Disease

- Depression affects approximately 50% of PD patients and accounts for the greatest impairment in quality of life
- The early stages of PD are commonly misdiagnosed as depression because of hypokinetic, cognitive, and neurovegetative symptoms
- Depression in PD presents primarily with anhedonia, anxiety, and sleep disturbances. Guilt, irritation, and psychotic features are uncommon
- An on/off phenomena may mimic depressive symptoms, but patients may respond acutely to levodopa

TREATMENT OF DEPRESSION IN PARKINSON'S DISEASE

- Management is complex because PD medications may cause psychiatric symptoms, but the treatment of these may in turn induce side effects that mimic PD (e.g., neuroleptic-induced EPS)
- Pramipexole (a D_2 and D_3 agonist used in PD) may be effective for depression in PD
- Selegiline (a type B MAOI) has not demonstrated antidepressant effects in PD
- SSRIs have not been studied in detail, but several reports have described an SSRI-induced exacerbation of motor symptoms
- TCAs (e.g., nortriptyline [≤150 mg/day], imipramine, and desipramine) have shown the best antidepressant effects in patients with PD. Elderly patients with PD should be monitored for TCA toxicity
- Selegiline is an MAOb inhibitor, and there have been rare reports of serotonin syndrome with TCAs and SSRIs
- ECT and transcranial magnetic stimulation (rTMS) over the dorsolateral prefrontal regions have shown antidepressant effects in PD patients and improvement of motor symptoms

Psychosis in Parkinson's Disease

- Psychotic symptoms occur in 20% to 30% of PD patients
- Psychotic symptoms may initially present as illusions or benign visual hallucinations and then progress to threatening hallucinations or paranoid delusions
- Predisposing factors: preexisting cognitive deterioration, psychiatric diseases, infection, medical illness, dehydration
- Both dopaminergic and anticholinergic medications for PD may induce psychosis

TREATMENT OF PSYCHOSIS OF PARKINSON'S DISEASE

- Rule out delirium (see page 9 for more information)
- Reduce or taper off PD drugs
- Reduce or discontinue anticholinergics, amantadine, and MAOIs
- Reduce or taper off dopamine agonists; then reduce levodopa
- Consider a course of antipsychotics:
  - Clozapine (50 mg): negligible risk for causing EPS; however, a weekly white blood cell (WBC) count must be obtained because of the risk of agranulocytosis
  - Quetiapine and olanzapine may also be used, although they have been reported to worsen EPS
  - Risperidone or typical antipsychotics should be used as a last resort

Other Neuropsychiatric Symptoms in Parkinson's Disease

- Dementia is common in patients with PD (see page 58 for more information)
- Increased libido and hypersexuality (particularly in men) may be seen after levodopa treatment
- Sleep disturbances (e.g., excessive daytime sleepiness, sleep attacks, and parasomnias): treat with sleep hygiene, nonbenzodiazepine hypnotics, or reduction of dopaminergic drugs (see page 97 for more information)
- OCD (see page 80 for more information)

Huntington's Disease (HD)

- **Definition:** Autosomal dominant neurodegenerative disorder characterized by progressive choreiform movements, ataxia, dementia, and neuropsychiatric symptoms
- **Symptoms:**
  - Behavioral symptoms are a hallmark of HD: irritability, bad temper, aggression, and agitation
  - Depression, anxiety, obsessions, compulsions, hallucinations, and delusions are very common and may precede the motor tics and choreiform movements
- There is a 12.7% rate of suicide and a high rate of alcohol abuse in patients with HD

Treatment of Huntington's Disease

- Primary goals: prevent self-harm and reduce symptoms
- Antipsychotics:
  - Effective in the management of chorea, tics, psychotic symptoms, and agitation
  - Small doses of haloperidol are useful early in the clinical course, but in later phases of the disease when EPS are more likely to appear, atypical antipsychotics (e.g., quetiapine and clozapine) are preferred

Multiple Sclerosis (MS)

- **Definition:** a chronic illness characterized by autoimmune-mediated demyelination of the CNS

- **Variable symptoms:** optic neuritis; diplopia; paresis; spasticity; ataxia; fatigue; heat sensitivity; cognitive impairment; Lhermitte's sign (flexion of the neck causing electric sensation down the spine); pain; bladder, bowel, and sexual dysfunction; hyperreflexia; internuclear ophthalmoplegia; psychiatric symptoms
- **Diagnosis:** lesions separated in time (two separate attacks or progression ≥6 mo) and space (multiple CNS locations); objective examination findings; no other disease to explain symptoms, magnetic resonance imaging findings (>9 lesions or ≥1 enhancing)
- **Course:** relapsing–remitting (35%), secondary progressive (45%), primary progressive (20%)
- **Psychiatric symptoms** are very common; as high as 90% of patients; include depression, elevated mood, and pseudobulbar affect (10%)
- **Depression:** high incidence (50% vs. 13% of rates among other chronic illnesses)
  - May develop at the onset of disease and may precede diagnosis
  - Higher rates of suicide
  - Increased risk of depression and mania with steroid treatment

SEIZURES

Symptoms

- Epilepsy: 1% lifetime prevalence
- Depression is common in patients with epilepsy (30%–50%)
- Suicide rate: five times greater than the general population (≤25 times higher in those with temporal lobe epilepsy)
- Psychosis: six to 12 times higher risk than the general population
  - Psychotic symptoms may be experienced during the aura, ictal, postictal, and interictal phases
  - Visual hallucinations in epilepsy: stereotyped, with or without aura, with or without postictal headache; duration is usually brief (a few seconds) vs. migraine visual symptoms, which have a longer duration
  - Occipital lobe seizures: characterized by brightly colored circles or that may change size, often in motion
  - Interictal personality change: hypergraphia, hyperreligiosity, hyposexuality, aggressivity, viscosity ("sticky, clingy")
- **Complex partial seizures** (most common in adults)
  - Temporal lobe epilepsy: aura with olfactory or other hallucinations, hyperreligiosity, macropsia, micropsia, déjà vu, jamais vu, dissociative symptoms, unprovoked panic
  - EEG may be negative in 40% of cases; a high index of suspicion must be maintained
  - Panic attacks may mimic partial complex seizures (although the postictal phase, impaired memory of event, and other stereotyped behaviors or perceptual disturbances are absent)

TABLE 4-25 Selected Differential Diagnosis of Nonconvulsive Seizures

Medical Conditions	Psychiatric Conditions
• Hypoglycemia • Migraine • Narcolepsy • Parasomnias • Transient ischemic attack	• Conversion disorder • Somatization • Dissociative disorder **Other** • Factitious disorder • Malingering

Adapted from Huffman J, Smith FA, Stern TA: Patients with neurologic conditions: seizure, cerebrovascular disease, and traumatic brain injury. In: Stern TA, Fricchione GL, Cassem NH, et al, eds. *Massachusetts General Hospital Handbook of General Hospital Psychiatry*, 5th ed. Philadelphia: Mosby; 2004:463.

Organ Failure and Transplantation

- Psychiatrists are often called to evaluate:
  - Agitation, delirium, or depression in patients with organ failure
  - Donor and recipient candidacy for organ transplantation
  - Mood disorders, compliance, complications of immunosuppression, chronic pain, substance abuse in posttransplant patients
- When evaluating patients with organ failure, be vigilant for delirium, adverse medication effects from drug–drug interactions, and compromised drug clearance

ORGAN FAILURE

Liver Failure

- **Definition:** liver dysfunction resulting in hepatic encephalopathy and impaired synthetic function (e.g., coagulopathy and hypoalbuminemia)
- Alcoholic cirrhosis and alcoholic hepatitis are most the common causes in the United States
- **Signs and symptoms of liver failure:**
  - GI: GI bleeds (upper GI bleeding, esophageal varices), ascites, pancreatitis, cirrhosis, hepatocellular carcinoma (from cirrhosis)
  - Neurologic: encephalopathy, asterixis, cognitive impairment
  - Renal: hepatorenal syndrome (renal failure from decreased renal perfusion)
  - Cardiovascular: hypotension, portal hypertension
  - Decreased synthetic function: coagulopathy, hypoalbuminemia
  - Infection: spontaneous bacterial peritonitis
  - Pulmonary: hepatopulmonary syndrome
  - "Stigmata of liver failure:" jaundice, spider angiomata, palmar erythema, gynecomastia, fetor hepaticus

Renal Failure

- **Acute renal failure:** acute deterioration in renal function as seen by increased creatinine
- **End-stage renal disease (ESRD):** failure of the kidneys to excrete wastes, concentrate urine, and regulate electrolytes
- **Common causes of chronic kidney disease:** hypertension, diabetes, polycystic kidney disease, glomerulonephritis, myeloma, lithium
- **Signs and symptoms of renal failure:**
  - Oliguria, increased creatinine, anemia, hyperkalemia (may lead to arrhythmia) acidosis, fluid overload, delirium, uremia (see below)
  - Hypocalcemia, hyperparathyroidism, hyperphosphatemia, vitamin D deficiency
- **Signs and symptoms of uremia:**
  - General: nausea, malaise, anorexia, pruritis, fetor uremicus
  - Neurologic: encephalopathy, seizures, myoclonus, neuropathy
  - Cardiovascular: pericarditis, congestive heart failure (CHF), volume overload, cardiomyopathy
  - Hematologic: bleeding (from platelet dysfunction), anemia
  - Metabolic: hyperkalemia, hyperphosphatemia, hypocalcemia, hyperparathyroidism, osteodystrophy

TREATMENT OF RENAL FAILURE

- Dialysis:
  - Access: AV fistula, AV graft, tunneled double-lumen catheter, temporary catheter
  - Common complications: hypotension (fluid shifts), heparin-induced thrombolysis, arrhythmia, sepsis (especially via access)
- Continuous venovenous hemofiltration
  - Used in critically ill patients; reduces fluid shifts
  - Complications: hypotension, infection, hypocalcemia, hypophosphatemia
- Peritoneal dialysis
  - Peritoneum acts as a membrane
  - Complications: peritonitis, hyperglycemia

Pulmonary Failure

- Causes of pulmonary failure: COPD, cystic fibrosis, pulmonary hypertension, idiopathic pulmonary fibrosis, α-1 antitrypsin deficiency

DETERMINING ORGAN TRANSPLANT CANDIDACY

Evaluation

- Major issues to consider when evaluating candidacy for organ transplantation:
  - Presence of active SI
  - Presence of major mood or thought disorders that may preclude the patient from following through with treatment
  - Presence of dementia (see page 58 for more information)
  - Active substance use (minimum requirement is usually 6 to 12 months of sustained sobriety)

- History of compliance with medications and treatment
- Presence of stable social supports
- Each transplant center has different criteria; consult your local guidelines

Psychiatric Symptoms Associated with Organ Failure and Transplantation

- Advanced medical illness and functional decline increase the risk for adjustment disorders, anxiety, and depression
- Organ failure and its treatment may also directly lead to anxiety, cognitive decline, and depression
- Posttransplant depressive symptoms (lethargy, appetite reduction, interpersonal withdrawal) may be early signs of infection (e.g., cytomegalovirus mycobacterium, *Listeria, Nocardia, Aspergillus*)
- New-onset psychiatric symptoms in the postoperative period should be prompt a workup for infection or other metabolic disturbances
- Pulmonary failure:
  - Shortness of breath is associated with anxiety
  - High frequency of panic attacks (panic disorder is as high as 17%)
  - Increased risk of delirium from hypoxia or hypercapnia
- Renal failure:
  - Depression is prevalent among patients with dialysis and may increase their mortality
  - Anemia and hyperparathyroidism may cause depression; fatigue, withdrawal, and apathy of uremia may be mistaken for depression (*continued*)

TABLE 4-26 Selected Differential Diagnosis of Psychiatric Symptoms with Organ Failure

Depression	• Anemia (especially in renal failure) • Fatigue • Hyperparathyroidism (e.g., in renal failure) • Hepatic encephalopathy • Infection: depression may herald infection in immunocompromised patients • Medications: interferon-α, immunosuppressants, opiates • Metabolic disturbances • Pain • Rejection of transplant, increase in cytokines • Uremia
Cognitive impairment	• Uremia, hepatic encephalopathy • Immunosuppressants • Delirium, hypoxia or hypercapnia • Dialysis dementia
Psychosis	• Steroid mania and psychosis • Infection • Seizure • Delirium

(*continued*)

- Liver failure:
  - Depression is common; also comorbid with alcohol dependence or hepatitis C virus coinfection
  - Comorbid substance abuse disorders should be actively treated
  - Hepatic encephalopathy may manifest as depressive symptoms, including withdrawal, apathy, anorexia, and subtle cognitive and behavioral changes

TABLE 4-27 Selected Differential Diagnosis of Delirium in Transplant Patients

- **Medication effects:** analgesics, anesthetics, immunosuppressant medications
- **Seizures:** associated with cyclosporine and tacrolimus
- **Steroids:** may cause agitation, mania, psychosis, sleep disturbance
- **Infection:** increased risk with immunosuppression
- **Toxicity:** from immunosuppressant drugs, increased risk with P450 inhibition
- **Withdrawal:** from alcohol, benzodiazepines, barbiturates, opiates
- **Intraoperative ischemia**
- **Metabolic abnormalities:** uremia, hyperammonemia, hyperkalemia, hyponatremia
- **Hemorrhage:** associated with uremia and coagulopathies

TABLE 4-28 Neuropsychiatric Side Effects of Transplantation Treatment

Cyclosporine (CYA; Sandimmune, Neoral)	Anxiety, psychosis, tremor, restlessness, seizures, leukoencephalopathy, hypomagnesemia, hyperkalemia, gastroparesis Toxic levels may lead to tremor, hypertension, nephrotoxicity, delirium
Mycophenolate (CellCept)	Anxiety and depression
Muromonab (OKT3)	Monoclonal antibody to treat rejection May cause tremor, delirium, seizures, and aseptic meningitis
Steroids	Insomnia, depression, anxiety, mania, psychosis, mood lability Dose related; increased risk with glucocorticoids
Tacrolimus (Prograf, FK506)	Insomnia, agitation, anxiety, headache At toxic levels, may lead to tremor, hypertension, renal dysfunction, delirium

Pharmacologic Treatment of Psychiatric Symptoms

- Assess whether the drug is hepatically or renally cleared
- Assess the degree of protein binding
- Be aware of accumulation of active metabolites when clearance is compromised
- Be aware of drug–drug interactions

SPECIFIC TREATMENT CONSIDERATIONS IN LIVER FAILURE

- See below for recommended dosage adjustments
- Benzodiazepines:
  - Use short-acting benzodiazepines
  - There is a high risk for obtundation and encephalopathy, so benzodiazepines should be used sparingly
  - Oxcarbazepam, temazepam, and lorazepam are preferred in patients with hepatic encephalopathy because first-pass oxidative metabolism is not required
- Antidepressants:
  - All carry small a risk of hepatotoxicity
  - Nefazodone has a black box warning for hepatoxicity
- Mood stabilizers: valproic acid is contraindicated in liver failure because of the risk of hyperammonemia

TABLE 4-29 Effects of Hepatic Failure on Selected Medications*

Medication	Standard Dosing (mg/day)	Recommended Dosing (mg/day)	Clinical Considerations
Alprazolam	0.75–5.0	0.375–5.00	Reduce dose by 50%
Bupropion	150–600	Reduced	Reduced dose and frequency; use extreme caution in patients with severe cirrhosis
Diazepam	4–40	2–20	Avoid in patients with severe and acute liver disease
Duloxetine	40–120	None	Not recommended in patients with any liver insufficiency
Fluoxetine	20–80	Reduced	Lower doses and increased interval between doses
Fluvoxamine	50–300	Reduced	Lower doses and increased interval between doses
Lithium	900–1200	Reduced	Use with caution, can be extremely difficult to dose
Paroxetine	20–60	10–30	50% reduction in daily dose
Quetiapine	50–800	May be reduced	Dose adjustment with hepatic insufficiency
Risperidone	1–10	1–4	Maximum dose of 2 mg BID is recommended with hepatic insufficiency
Sertraline	50–200	50–200	Initial dose <50 mg or increase dosing interval >24 hrs
Valproate	15–60/kg	None	Contraindicated in patients with hepatic failure

* This table is not comprehensive. Clinicians should evaluate all medications in patients with renal disease and follow guidelines set by the manufacturer in all prescribing decisions.
BID, twice a day.

SPECIFIC TREATMENT CONSIDERATIONS FOR RENAL FAILURE

- See below for recommended dosage reductions
- Benzodiazepines: choose short-acting drugs to minimize buildup of metabolites
- Mood stabilizers:
  - Follow free or unbound levels whenever possible (shifts in protein binding make interpreting some blood levels difficult)
  - Lithium: give after dialysis because it is easily dialyzed

MISCELLANEOUS PHARMACOLOGIC CONCERNS IN TRANSPLANT PATIENTS

- Phenytoin and phenobarbital may decrease immunosuppressant levels
- Lithium: use care because of an increased risk of toxicity with cyclosporine
- Cyclosporine levels are decreased by valproic acid, carbamazepine, and phenobarbital

TABLE 4-30 Effects of Renal Failure on Selected Medications*

Medication	Standard Dosing (mg/day)	Recommended Dosing (mg/day)	Clinical Considerations
Chlordiazepoxide	15–100	7.5–50	Decreased protein binding and increased clearance in renal disease
Lithium	900–1200	200–600	Administration of a single dose after dialysis is recommended
Lorazepam	3–6 mg (BID or TID dosing)	0.5–2.0 (BID dosing)	Not recommended for use in ESRD by manufacturer
Mirtazapine	15–45	7.5–22.5	Clearance reduced ~50% in renal disease
Paroxetine	20–60	10–30	Decreased metabolism possibly because of CYP2D6 inhibition
Valproate	15–60/kg	15–60/kg	Increased free serum levels in ESRD Use free valproic acid levels when monitoring
Risperidone	1–3 (BID dosing)	0.5–1.5	Clearance reduced by 60% in ESRD
Zolpidem	10	5	Increased free fraction in renal disease

*This table is not comprehensive. Clinicians should evaluate all medications in patients with renal disease and follow guidelines set by the manufacturer in all prescribing decisions.
BID, twice a day; ESRD, end-stage renal disease; TID, three times a day.

Culture and Psychiatry

- Culture affects illness presentation, access to care, diagnosis, and treatment
- This section addresses:
  - Evaluation and treatment of a patient from a different culture
  - Working with interpreters
  - Culture-bound syndromes
  - Ethnicity and psychopharmacology
  - Disparities

TABLE 4-31 Approach to the Evaluation of Culturally Diverse Patients

General Considerations
• Ask about the patient's cultural identity (don't assume) • Explore the link between symptoms and cultural influences (don't assume that general cultural beliefs apply to individual cases) • Explore the meaning of an illness in relation to the patient's culture, family, and community • Inquire about herbal and spiritual remedies
Interview Tips
• Address the patient formally at the initial meeting because people in some cultures interpret informal introductions as disrespectful (Henderson, 2007) • Ask the least intrusive questions early in the interview because people in many cultures have strong negative stigma regarding the mental health profession
Basic Questions
• What languages do you speak? Would you like an interpreter? • Where are you from originally? • Immigration questions: ask "who, when, where, what, why" did you leave your country of origin? • Immigration status? • Exposure to violence and trauma?

USING AN INTERPRETER

- Avoid using family members as interpreters
- Avoid two-way conversations either between the interpreter and patient or the interpreter and clinician
- Discuss the expectations and goals of the patient encounter with the interpreter
- Introduce the interpreter at the beginning of the session and reaffirm patient confidentiality
- Speak directly to the patient
- Maintain eye contact with the patient
- Speak slowly
- Use short sentences and avoid medical jargon
- Meet with the interpreter after the session to obtain clarification and feedback
- Interpreter services:
  - 1-800-translate.com
  - languageline.com
  - http://www.usa.att.com
  - certifiedlanguages.com
  - languagefon.com.

Please note that these services may charge a fee

CULTURE-SPECIFIC PSYCHIATRIC CONCERNS

Cultural Differences in Presentation of Illness

- Somatic symptoms may be the only indication of depression in certain cultures
- Psychotic symptoms may be difficult to distinguish from culturally normative traditions (e.g., hearing voices of ancestors, communicating with spirits, belief in witchcraft)
- Bias in diagnosis and treatment: African American patients are more likely to be misdiagnosed with schizophrenia and given higher doses of antipsychotic agents
- *DSM* diagnoses may not be valid in other cultures or societies

Culture-Bound Syndromes

- Culture-bound syndromes describe recurrent, locality-specific illnesses that may or may not relate to particular *DSM-IV-TR* categories
- Selected common culture-bound syndromes are listed below

Amok (Malaysia)

- A dissociative episode of violent or homicidal behavior that is provoked by a perceived insult. Occurs in males and may be associated with psychotic episodes

Ataque de nervios (Caribbean, widespread Latino cultures)

- An expression of distress that often occurs after a stressful family event. Distress is manifested as out-of-control shouting, trembling, and crying. It may also be expressed as agitation, aggression, or a sensation of heat in the chest rising into the head

Bilis and colera (also referred to as muina; Latino cultures)

- Anger or rage that manifests as acute nervousness, tension, trembling, and screaming. Also associated with headache, stomach disturbances, and even loss of consciousness

Bouffée delirante (West Africa and Haiti)

- A syndrome of acute-onset agitation and aggression, confusion, and psychomotor excitement. May also present with hallucinations or paranoia; resembles brief psychotic disorder

Ghost sickness (various American Indian tribes)

- A fixation with death and those who are dead. Symptoms include weakness, syncope, hallucinations, nightmares, hopelessness, confusion, and anorexia

Koro (South and East Asia)

- Belief that the penis will disappear into the body, possibly causing death. In women, the belief involves the nipples and vulva

Latah (Malaysia and Indonesia)

- Hypersensitivity to sudden fright. Symptoms include echopraxia, echolalia, command obedience, and dissociative behavior

Mal de Ojo (widespread)

- "Evil eye." Symptoms include crying episodes, disrupted sleep, diarrhea, vomiting, or fever in children

Ethnopsychopharmacology

- Understanding how both pharmacokinetics and environmental factors relate to different populations helps practitioners predict side effects, blood levels, and potential drug–drug interactions
- Genetic variation of enzymes in the P450 system that metabolize psychotropic drugs leads to differences in side effects, toxicity, and efficacy
- Poor metabolizers (individuals with decreased enzyme activity) are at a greater risk for toxicity and side effects, even at low medication doses

TABLE 4-32 Enzyme Status Across Different Populations

2D6	2C19
• Metabolizes most antidepressants (SSRIs, TCAs, heterocyclics) and antipsychotics (e.g., Haldol, clozapine) • Incidence of "poor metabolizers": • 3%–7% in whites • 0%–18% in African Americans • 0.5%–2.4% in Asians • 4.5% in Hispanics	• Metabolizes diazepam, clomipramine, imipramine, propranolol • The incidence of "poor metabolizers" of this enzyme are in the range of: • 3%–5% in whites • 4%–18% in African Americans • 18%–23% in Asians (Henderson, 2006; Lin, 1983)

SSRI, selective serotonin reuptake inhibitor; TCA, tricyclic antidepressant.
Adapted from Henderson DC, Nguyen DD, Vuky C: The importance of culture. In: Stern TA, ed. *The Ten-Minute Guide to Psychiatric Diagnosis and Treatment.* New York: Professional Publishing Group; 2005:447–462.

Considerations when Prescribing Psychotropic Medications

- Asians have been shown to have up to 50% greater blood levels of certain antipsychotic medications than white patients
- Asians have higher rates of EPS and respond to lower levels of clozapine, lithium, and benzodiazepines
- African Americans may have a greater risk of neurotoxicity from TCAs and lithium
- African Americans have much higher incidences of hypertension, obesity, diabetes, and DKA

Disparities

- A growing body of evidence shows that minorities receive lower quality of mental health care, are prescribed drugs differently (e.g., less likely to receive SSRIs or second-generation antipsychotics), and have less money spent on their care

REFERENCES

CHILDREN AND ADOLESCENTS

Centers for Disease Control and Prevention. Suicide trends among youths and young adults aged 10–24 years—United States, 1990–2004. *MMWR Morb Mortal Wkly Rep* 2007;56(35):905–908.

Hartman RG. Adolescent decisional autonomy for medical care: physician perceptions and practices. *University of Chicago Law School Roundtable* 2001;8:87.

Hussey JM, Chang JJ, Kotch JB: Child maltreatment in the United States: prevalence, risk factors, and adolescent health consequences. *Pediatrics* 2006;118(3): 933–942.

Johnston LD, O'Malley PM, Bachman JG, et al. *Monitoring the Future National Survey Results on Drug Use, 1975–2007. Volume 1: Secondary School Students.* NIH Publication No. 08-6418A. Bethesda, MD: National Institute on Drug Abuse; 2008.

Petit J. *Handbook of Emergency Psychiatry.* Philadelphia: Lippincott Williams & Wilkins; 2004:265–270.

Prager L, Schlozman S, Jellinek M. Affective disorders and suicide. In: Rudolph CD, ed. *Rudolph's Pediatrics* New York McGraw-Hill; in press.

WOMEN

Chaudron LH, Pies RW. The relationship between postpartum psychosis and bipolar disorder: a review. *J Clin Psychiatry* 2003;64(11):1284–1292.

Han E, Liu GG. Racial disparities in prescription drug use for mental illness among population in US. *J Ment Health Policy Econ* 2005;8(3):131–143.

Joffe H, Cohen LS, Suppes T, et al. Valproate is associated with new-onset oligoamenorrhea with hyperandrogenism in women with bipolar disorder. *Biol Psychiatry* 2006;1;59(11):1078–86.

Massachusetts General Hospital Center for Women's Health. *Reproductive Psychiatry Resource and Information Center.* Available at: http://www.womensmentalhealth.org.

National Institute of Mental Health: *Women and Mental Health.* Available at: http://www.nimh.nih.gov/health/topics/women-and-mental-health/index.shtml.

GERIATRIC PATIENTS

Alexopoulos GS. Depression in the elderly. *Lancet* 2005;365(9475):1961–1970.

Cremens MC. Care of the geriatric patient. In: Stern TA, Fricchione GL, Cassem NH, et al, eds. *Massachusetts General Hospital Handbook of General Hospital Psychiatry,* 5th ed. Philadelphia: Mosby; 2004:447–456.

Inouye SK. Delirium in older persons. *N Engl J Med* 2006;354(11):1157–1165.

Rosenberg PB, Johnston D, Lyketsos CG: A clinical approach to mild cognitive impairment. *Am J Psychiatry* 2006;163(11):1884–1890.

Rinaldi P, Mecocci P, Benedetti C, et al. Validation of the five-item geriatric depression scale in elderly subjects in three different settings. *J Am Geriatr Soc* 2003;51(5): 694–698.

MEDICALLY ILL PATIENTS

Alpert JE, Fava M, Rosenbaum JF. Pharmacologic issues in the medical setting. In: Stern TA, Fricchione GL, Cassem NH, et al, eds. *Massachusetts General Hospital Handbook of General Hospital Psychiatry,* 5th ed. Philadelphia: Mosby; 2004: 231–269.

Beck BJ. An approach to the diagnosis and treatment of mental disorders in the context of a general medical condition. In: Stern T, ed. *The Ten-Minute Guide to Psychiatric Diagnosis and Treatment.* New York: Professional Publishing; 2005: 75–97.

Beck BJ: Mental disorders due to a general medical condition. In: Stern, TA, Rosenbaum JR, Fava M, et al, eds. *Massachusetts General Hospital Comprehensive Clinical Psychiatry.* Philadelphia: Mosby Elsevier; 2008:257–281.

Heckers S, Pasinksi RC. The patient with neuropsychiatric dysfunction. In: Stern TA, Herman JB, Slavin PL, eds. *Massachusetts General Hospital Guide to Primary Care Psychiatry,* 2nd ed. New York: McGraw-Hill; 2004:216–222.

Huffman JC, Stern TA. Side effects of psychotropic medications. In: Stern TA, Rosenbaum JR, Fava M, et al, eds. *Massachusetts General Hospital Comprehensive Clinical Psychiatry.* Philadelphia: Mosby Elsevier; 2008:705–720.

Iosifescu DV. Treating depression in the medically ill. *Psychiatr Clin North Am* 2007;30(1):77–90.

Rosenbaum JF, Arana GW, Hyman SE, et al, eds. *Handbook of Psychiatric Drug Therapy,* 5th ed. Philadelphia: Lippincott Williams & Wilkins; 2005.

Smith FS, Wittmann CW, Stern TA. Medical complications of psychiatric treatment. *Critical Care Clin* 2008; in press.

CANCER

Greenberg DB, Pirl WF. Cancer. In: Stern TA, Rosenbaum JR Fava M, et al, eds. *Massachusetts General Hospital Comprehensive Clinical Psychiatry.* Philadelphia: Mosby Elsevier; 2008:773–787.

Milovic M, Block S. Psychiatric disorders in advanced cancer. *Cancer* 2007;110:1665–1676.

CARDIAC ILLNESS

Barth J, Schumacher MA, Herrmann-Lingen C. Depression as a risk factor for mortality in patients with coronary heart disease: a meta-analysis. *Psychosom Med* 2004;66: 802–813.

Frasure-Smith N, Lesperance F. Depression and anxiety as predictors of 2-year cardiac events in patients with stable coronary artery disease. *Arch Gen Psychiatry* 2008; 65:62.

Glassman AH, O'Connor CM, Califf RM, et al. Sertraline treatment of major depression in patients with acute MI or unstable angina. *JAMA* 2002;288:701–709.

Huffman JC, Stern TA. Neuropsychiatric consequences of cardiovascular medications. *Dialogues Clin Neurosci* 2007;9:57–73.

Huffman JC, Stern TA, Januzzi JL. The psychiatric management of patients with cardiac disease. In: Stern TA, Fricchione GL, Cassem NH, et al, eds. *Massachusetts General Handbook of General Hospital Psychiatry.* Philadelphia: Mosby; 2004:547–569.

Lespérance F, Frasure-Smith N, Koszycki D, et al. Effects of citalopram and interpersonal psychotherapy on depression in patients with coronary artery disease: the Canadian Cardiac Randomized Evaluation of Antidepressant and Psychotherapy Efficacy (CREATE) trial. *JAMA* 2007;297:367–379.

Serebruany VL, Suckow RF, Cooper TB, et al. Relationship between release of platelet/endothelial biomarkers and plasma levels of sertraline and N-desmethylsertraline in acute coronary syndrome patients receiving SSRI treatment for depression. *Am J Psychiatry,* 2005;162:1165–1170.

HIV/AIDS PSYCHIATRY

Bartlett JG. *The Johns Hopkins Hospital 2004–2005 Guide to Medical Care of Patients with HIV Infection,* 12th ed. Philadelphia, PA: Lippincott Williams & Wilkins; 2005.

Body Health Resources Corporation. *The BodyPRO.* Available at: http://www.thebodypro.com.

Centers for Disease Control and Prevention. *HIV/AIDS.* Available at: http://www.cdc.gov/hiv.

Johns Hopkins Hospital. *HIV Guide.* Available at: http://www.hopkins-aids.edu.

Power C, Selnes OA, Grim JA, et al. HIV dementia scale: a rapid screening test. *J Acquir Immune Defic Syndr Hum Retrovirol* 1995;8(3):273–278.

Querques J, Freudenreich O. HIV and AIDS. In: Stern TA, Rosenblum JF, Fava M, et al, eds. *Massachusetts General Hospital Comprehensive Clinical Psychiatry.* Philadelphia: Mosby; 2008:787–802.

US Department of Health and Human Services. *AIDSinfo.* Available at: http://www.aidsinfo.nih.gov.

NEUROLOGIC ILLNESS

Cantello R, Gilli M, Riccio A, et al. Mood changes associated with "end-dose deterioration" in Parkinson's disease. *J Neurol Neurosurg Psychiatr* 1986;49:1190.

Carson AJ, MacHale S, Allen K, et al. Depression after stroke and lesion location: a systematic review. *Lancet* 2000;356(9224):122–126.

Huffman JC, Smith, FA, Stern, TA, et al. Patients with neurological conditions. In: Stern TA, Fricchione GL, Cassem NH, et al, eds. *Massachusetts General Hospital Handbook of General Hospital Psychiatry,* 5th ed. Philadelphia: Mosby; 2004:457–473.

Kaufman D. *Clinical Neurology for Psychiatrists.* Philadelphia: WB Saunders; 2001.

Kuzuhara S. Drug-induced psychotic symptoms in Parkinson's disease. *J Neurol* 200; 248(suppl 3):28–31.

Roffman JL, Eisenberg T, Stern TA. Neuropsychiatric phenomena associated with movement disorders. *Prim Care Companion J Clin Psychiatry* 2006;8(1):39-42.

Starkstein SE, Robinson RG. Stroke. In: Coffey CE, Cummings JL, eds. *The American Psychiatric Press Textbook of Geriatric Neuropsychiatry.* Washington, DC: American Psychiatric Publishing; 2000:601–620.

ORGAN FAILURE AND TRANSPLANTATION

Cohen LM, Tessier EG, Germain MJ, et al. Update on psychotropic medication use in renal disease. *Psychosomatics* 2004;45:1.

Crone CC, Gabriel GM, DiMartini A. An overview of psychiatric issues in liver disease for the consultation-liaison psychiatrist. *Psychosomatics* 2006;47:188–205.

Prager L. Organ transplantation. In: Stern, TA, Rosenbaum JR, Fava M, et al, eds. *Massachusetts General Hospital Comprehensive Clinical Psychiatry.* Philadelphia: Mosby; 2008.

Sabatine M. Pocket Medicine. In: *The Massachusetts General Hospital Handbook of Internal Medicine,* 2nd ed. Philadelphia: Lippincott; 2004.

Surman O, Prager L. Organ failure and transplantation. In: Stern TA, Fricchione GL, Cassem NH, et al, eds. *The Massachusetts General Hospital Handbook of General Hospital Psychiatry,* 5th ed. Philadelphia: Mosby; 2004:641–669.

CULTURE AND PSYCHIATRY

American Psychiatric Association. *Diagnostic and Statistical Manual of Mental Disorders,* 4th ed, text rev. Washington, DC: American Psychiatric Association; 2000.

Henderson DC, Nguyen DD, Vuky C. The importance of culture. In: Stern TA, ed. *The Ten-Minute Guide to Psychiatric Diagnosis and Treatment.* New York: Professional Publishing Group; 2005:447–462.

Henderson DC, Yeung A, Xiaoduo F, et al. Culture and psychiatry. In: Stern TA, ed. *The Ten-Minute Guide to Psychiatric Diagnosis and Treatment.* New York: Professional Publishing Group; 2005:737–748.

Henderson DC. Atypical antipsychotic-induced diabetes mellitus: how strong is the evidence? *CNS Drugs* 2002;16(2):77–89.

Lim RF. *Clinical Manual of Cultural Psychiatry.* Washington, DC: American Psychiatric Publishing; 2006:207–240.

Lin KM. Psychopharmacology in cross-cultural psychiatry. *Mt Sinai J Med* 1996;63(5–6): 283–284.

Lin TY. Psychiatry and Chinese culture. *West J Med* 1983;139(6):862–867.

Lu FG, Lim RF, Mezzich JE. Issues in the assessment and diagnosis of culturally diverse individuals. In: Oldham JM, Riba MB, eds. *American Psychiatric Press Review of Psychiatry*, vol 14. Washington, DC: American Psychiatric Press; 1995:477–510.

Marcos LR, Cancro R. Pharmacotherapy of Hispanic depressed patients: clinical observations. *Am J Psychother* 1982;36:505–513.

Silver B, Poland RE, Lin KM. Ethnicity and the pharmacology of tricyclic antidepressants. In: Lin KM, Poland RE, Nakasaki G, eds. *Psychopharmacology and Psychobiology of Ethnicity*. Washington, DC, American Psychiatric Press; 1993:61–89.

Wagner GJ, Maguen S, Rabkin JG. Ethnic differences in response to fluoxetine in a controlled trial with depressed HIV-positive patients. *Psychiatr Serv* 1998;49: 239–240.

The Organization of Student Representatives. Guidelines for the use of medical interpreter services. *AAMC* 2006.

Chapter 5

TREATMENT MODALITIES

PSYCHOPHARMACOLOGIC AGENTS

1. Food and Drug Administration (FDA) pharmaceutical pregnancy classification
2. Receptors targeted by psychopharmacologic agents
3. Pharmacologic treatment of depression
   a. Names and doses of commonly used agents
   b. Selective serotonin reuptake inhibitors (SSRIs) and serotonin and norepinephrine reuptake inhibitors (SNRIs)
   c. Tricyclic antidepressants (TCAs) and monoamine oxidase inhibitors (MAOIs)
   d. Alternative agents
4. Pharmacologic treatment of anxiety
   a. Agents used to treat anxiety
5. Pharmacologic treatment of bipolar disorder
   a. Evidence of efficacy of selected agents
   b. Names and doses of commonly used agents
   c. Specific characteristics of:
      i. Lithium
      ii. Valproate
      iii. Carbamazepine
      iv. Lamotrigine
6. Pharmacologic treatment of psychosis
   a. "Typical" (first-generation) neuroleptics
   b. "Atypical" (second-generation) antipsychotics
   c. Clozapine
7. Medications used in the treatment of dementia
   a. Names and doses of commonly used agents
   b. Anticholinesterase and N-methyl-D-aspartic acid (NMDA)agents
8. Medications used in the treatment of attention-deficit hyperactivity disorder (ADHD)
   a. Names and doses of commonly used agents
   b. Summary of properties of stimulants
9. Medications used for treatment of substance dependence and withdrawal
   a. Alcohol
   b. Nicotine
   c. Opiates
10. Sedative–hypnotics and other sedating drugs
11. Proposed herbal remedies for psychiatric symptoms
12. Common adverse effects and their management
13. Somatic Therapies
14. Psychotherapies

TABLE 5-1 Food and Drug Administration Pharmaceutical Pregnancy Classification

- **Category A:** Adequate and well-controlled studies have failed to demonstrate a risk to the fetus in the first trimester of pregnancy (and there is no evidence of risk in later trimesters)
- **Category B:** animal reproduction studies have failed to demonstrate a risk to the fetus, and there are no adequate and well-controlled studies in pregnant women OR animal studies have shown an adverse effect, but adequate and well-controlled studies in pregnant women have failed to demonstrate a risk to the fetus in any trimester
- **Category C:** animal reproduction studies have shown an adverse effect on the fetus and there are no adequate and well-controlled studies in humans, but potential benefits may warrant use of the drug in pregnant women despite potential risks
- **Category D:** there is positive evidence of human fetal risk based on adverse reaction data from investigational or marketing experience or studies in humans, but potential benefits may warrant use of the drug in pregnant women despite potential risks
- **Category X:** studies in animals or humans have demonstrated fetal abnormalities and/or there is positive evidence of human fetal risk based on adverse reaction data from investigational or marketing experience, and the risks involved in use of the drug in pregnant women clearly outweigh the potential benefits

PHARMACOLOGIC TREATMENT OF DEPRESSION

Choosing an Agent

- See p. 65 for a general discussion of diagnosis and treatment
- Clinical outcomes, quality-of-life outcomes, and cost analyses provide minimal guidance
- Initial choice should be based on adverse effects, interactions with other medications, and tolerability

Dosages

- Start at a low dose and titrate gradually in elderly patients, and provide adequate milligrams per kilograms in children
- Increase the dose after 1 to 2 weeks
- Doses may need to be higher with chronic illness or comorbid conditions (e.g., anxiety)

Monitoring

- Follow-up visits should be done twice or month or more for several months, especially with severely depressed or suicidal patients
- Monitor adherence to prescribed treatment

Changing and Augmenting Therapy

- Can switch medications (to same or different class) or supplement with adjunctive medication if there has been no response by 8 to 12 weeks at a maximal dose
- Typical augmentation strategies include lithium, lamotrigine, other anticonvulsants, buspirone, stimulants, low doses of atypical antipsychotics (e.g., quetiapine), and natural supplements (*continued*)

TABLE 5-2 Receptors Targeted by Psychopharmacologic Agents

Class and Receptors Affected	Relevant Transporters and Clearance Mechanisms	CNS Targets	Actions	Agonists	Antagonists	Functional Pathways
Dopamine (DA) D2 D4	↓DAT ↓MAO	**DA neurons** in nigro-striatal, mesolimbic and tuberoin-fundibular circuits **D2: DA** cell bodies, terminals; lactotrophs (anterior pituitary) **D4:** frontal cortex, medulla, midbrain (VTA)	**D2, D4:** ↓AC, ↓cAMP, ↑K+, ↓C^- conductance **DAT:** Na^+/K^+ pump, clears DA from synaptic cleft **MAO:** catabolizes monoamines	**D2:** bromocriptine, pramipexole **DAT:** Bupropion and Wellbutrin (?), amphetamines (increase DA-release), methylphenidate (blocks reuptake) **MAO:** MAOIs	**D2:** typical and atypical antipsychotics **D4:** atypical antipsychotics	Cognition Motor activity Motivation and reward Prolactin production (inhibitory) Sleep Mood Attention and learning
Norepinephrine (NE) α_1 α_2	↓SERT ↓MAO	Neurons originate mostly in the locus ceruleus and innervate the forebrain and cerebellum	α_1: ↑IP_3 DAG/Ca^{2+} α_2: ↓AC, ↓cAMP, ↑K^+, ↑Cl^- (autoreceptor) **NET:** Na^+/Cl^- driven NE transporter, clears NE **MAO:** catabolizes monoamines	**NET:** SNRIs, NRIs, TCAs, bupropion (block reuptake), amphetamines (increase release of NE) α_2: clonidine (agonist), mirtazapine (antagonizes and increases release of NE, 5HT) MAO: MAOIs	**NET:** trazodone α_1: TCAs, low-potency typical antipsychotics, trazodone, atypical antipsychotics	Arousal Attention Vasopressin

Serotonin (5-OH-tryptamine, 5HT) $5HT_{1A,B,D,E,F}$ $5HT_{2A,B,C}$ $5HT_3$ $5HT_{4,6,7}$	↓SERT ↓MAO	**$5HT_{1A}$:** limbic: postsynaptic, raphe **$5HT_{2A}$:** cortex **$5HT_{2C}$:** widespread **$5HT_3$:** hippocampus, solitary tract, postrema **$5HT_5$:** hypothalamus, corpus callosum, ventricles **$5HT_6$:** striatum, limbic areas, cortex **$5HT_7$:** cortex, thalamus, midbrain, raphe NN; SERT (reuptake): pre-synaptic cortical, neostriatum, thalamus, limbic	**$5HT_{1A,B,D,E,F}$:** ↓AC,↓cAMP, activates K^+ channels **$5HT_{2A,B,C}$:** ↑IP_3/DAG/Ca^{2+} **$5HT_3$:** ligand-gated Na+ channel **$5HT_{4,5,6,7}$:** ↑AC, ↑cAMP **5HTT:** Na^+/K^+ ATPase-dependent, clears 5HT **MAO:** catabolizes monoamines (NE, 5HT, DA)	**$5HT_{1A}$:** buspirone/BuSpar (partial), TCAs (upregulate) **$5HT_2$:** TCAs (downregulate) **$5HT_{2aA2C}$:** trazodone (downregulate) **$5HT_{2/3}$:** mirtazapine/Remeron (antagonist) **5-HTT:** SRIs, SNRIs, TCAs, trazodone/Desyrel **SRIs** (block reuptake)	**$5HT_{1A}$:** buspirone **$5HT_2$:** atypical antipsychotics, trazodone **$5HT_{2A/2C/3}$:** mirtazapine	Mood Sleep Aggression Appetite Metabolism Sexuality Anger Vomiting

5HT, serotonin; AC, adenylyl cyclase; AChE, acetylcholinesterase; cAMP, cyclic adenosine monophosphate; CNS, central nervous system DA, dopamine; DAG, diacylglycerol; DAT, dopamine transporter; IP_3, inositol-1,4,5-triphosphate; mACh, muscarinic acetylcholine; MAO, monoamine oxidase; MAOIs, monoamine oxidase inhibitors; NE, norepinephrine; NET, norepinephrine transporter; NRI, norepinephrine reuptake inhibitor; PLC, phospholipase C; SERT: serotonin transporter; SNRI, serotonin and norepinephrine reuptake inhibitor; SRI, serotonin reuptake inhibitor; TCA: tricyclic and tetracyclic antidepressant.

TABLE 5-3 Amino Acids and Other Transmitters

Class and Receptors Affected	CNS Targets	Actions	Agonists	Antagonists
GABA, $GABA_A$	Limbic, cortical areas	**$GABA_A$: ↑Cl^-** conductance (hyperpolarizes)	**$GABA_A$:** Benzodiazepines (BZ_1 or BZ_2 receptors); other hypnotics	
Glutamate, NMDA	NMDA in cortex, hippocampus, striatum, septum, amygdala	**NMDA:** inotropic: ↑Na^+, ↑Ca^{2+}, ↑CaMKII		**NMDA:** memantine/ Namenda
Histamine/ H1	Tuberomammillary neurons to forebrain	**H1: ↑IP3/** DAG/Ca2$^+$	**H_1:** (e.g., mirtazapine, doxepin)	**H_1:** TCAs, mirtazapine, trazodone, low-potency typical antipsychotics, antihistamines (diphenhydramine)
Melatonin/ MT_1, MT_2	From suprachiasmatic nucleus		**MT_1, MT_2 agonists** (e.g., ramelteon)	

DAG, diacylglycerol; GABA, γ-aminobutyric acid; IP_3: inositol-1,4,5-triphosphate; NMDA, N-methyl-D-aspartic acid; TCA, tricyclic and tetracyclic antidepressant.

(*continued*)

Maintenance

- The goal should be complete remission of symptoms
- Continue for at least 6 months, even after recovery

Cessation

- Early withdrawal and discontinuation syndromes can occur within days after rapid discontinuation of short-acting agents
  - SSRIs and SNRIs: may include dizziness, nausea, fatigue, muscle aches, chills, anxiety, irritability
  - TCAs: irritability, agitation, sleep disturbance, flu-like symptoms, cardiac arrhythmia (rare)

- MAOIs: delirium, agitation, myoclonic jerks, insomnia
- Bupropion, fluoxetine, mirtazapine: uncommon
- Continuation of MAOI effects after cessation may interact with other agents and foods to induce delirium and death (SSRIs, meperidine, tyramine in foods)
- Rapid discontinuation of antidepressant can lead to increased risk of relapse, sometimes with more severe depression than in past
- Reducing doses slowly over 2 to 4 weeks of medications with short half-lives may reduce the risk of early and later adverse outcomes

Pregnancy

- All antidepressants are category C (some animal studies show adverse effects, but no controlled studies in humans are available) or D (there is evidence of risk to human fetuses, but the potential benefits may justify the risk)
- Consider cognitive behavioral therapy (CBT), interpersonal therapy, supportive therapy, electroconvulsive therapy (ECT), and hospitalization when medications are contraindicated

TABLE 5-4 Pharmacologic Agents For Depression (Food and Drug Administration Approved and Off Label)

Drug Type	Actions	Therapeutics	Limitations, Contraindications, and Side Effects
Selective serotonin reuptake inhibitors	Block reuptake of 5HT at SERT	Common initial treatment Nonlethal in overdose Generally mild adverse effects Low doses may work for panic and anxiety disorders, but, patients with OCD require high doses	May lead to weight gain, agitation, insomnia or sedation GI and sexual side effects common Discontinuation syndrome with drugs that have short half-life (e.g., paroxetine)
Serotonin norepinephrine reuptake inhibitors	Block reuptake of 5HT and NE at both SERT and NET sites	FDA indication for depression Duloxetine, high doses of venlafaxine, or tertiary-amine TCAs may be used for neuropathic pain	Liver disease: duloxetine is contraindicated High blood pressure: venlafaxine is contraindicated Duloxetine: relatively dangerous in overdose Early discontinuation syndrome is common with venlafaxine

(continued)

TABLE 5-4 Pharmacologic Agents For Depression (Food and Drug Administration Approved and Off Label) (*continued*)

Drug Type	Actions	Therapeutics	Limitations, Contraindications, and Side Effects
Bupropion (Wellbutrin, Zyban)	Weakly blocks uptake of DA and NE at DAT and NET sites	Adverse sexual effects are rare May be stimulating Often useful as an SRI adjunct Help with smoking cessation	May lower the seizure threshold at higher doses and perhaps with bulimia or alcohol-dependence
Mirtazapine (Remeron)	Agonist at α_2 adrenergic and 5HT-2a, -2C, -3 auto, and other receptors to facilitate release of both NE and 5-HT Blocks H1 receptors (sedating)	Moderate sexual adverse effects Useful for patients with insomnia or anorexia	May cause weight-gain, sedation, autonomic effects, or rare neutropenia (monitor CBC)
Tricyclic agents (TCAs: amitriptyline, clomipramine, desipramine, doxepin, imipramine, nortriptyline, protriptyline, trimipramine)	Block reuptake of 5HT and NE if tertiary-amines (amitriptyline), but mainly NE if secondary amines (desipramine)	Now held as a secondary option for otherwise resistant depression Often reduce tics Overdoses can be lethal (cardiotoxicity and delirium)	Contraindicated with glaucoma, past MI, diabetes Risks: weight-gain, GI symptoms, urinary retention, confusion in elderly patients
Monoamine oxidase inhibitors (phenelzine, selegiline, tranylcypromine)	Prolonged anti-MAO-A and B actions Selegiline has some MAO-B selectivity at low doses (safer with sympatho-mimetics), but MAO-A inhibition is more antidepressant	Third-line treatment for resistant depression Autonomic and sexual effects mimic those of the anticholinergics	Dietary restrictions to avoid tyramine and other sympathomimetics Many drug interactions (especially SSRIs and methylphenidate) May be lethal in overdose

(*continued*)

TABLE 5-4 Pharmacologic Agents For Depression (Food and Drug Administration Approved and Off Label) (*continued*)

Drug Type	Actions	Therapeutics	Limitations, Contraindications, and Side Effects
Lamotrigine Lamictal)	Blocks voltage-sensitive Na^+-channels, inhibits release of excitatory amino acids glutamate and aspartate	Increase the dose slowly and monitor to avoid adverse effects (skin toxicity: dose and rate dependent, worse with valproate); restart at original dose if discontinued >4 days	May cause mild (common) or severe (rare) rash and blood dyscrasias
Quetiapine (Seroquel)	Atypical antipsychotic, serotonin/dopamine antagonist; strongly anti-H_1 (sedative) Metabolite may block NET	Helpful for patients with anxiety and insomnia (low doses) or psychosis (high doses)	Weight gain, sedation, orthostatic hypotension
Atomoxetine (NRI, Strattera)	Mainly a NET inhibitor	Weakly effective in patients with ADHD	Not clearly effective in MDD
Stimulants (methylphenidate, amphetamines)	Mainly release and prevent reuptake of DA and NE	Used in treatment-resistant depression and in elderly patients to assist with appetite and energy	Potential for abuse May induce mania in bipolar disorder (as can all antidepressants as doses increase) May worsen OCD and induce tics

5HT, serotonin; ADHD, attention-deficit hyperactivity disorder; CBC, complete blood count; DA, dopamine; DAT, dopamine transporter; GI, gastrointestinal; MAO, monoamine oxidase; MDD, major depressive disorder; MI, myocardial infarction; NE, norepinephrine; NET, norepinephrine transporter; NRI, norepinephrine reuptake inhibitor; OCD, obsessive–compulsive disorder; SERT, serotonin transporter; SSRI, selective serotonin reuptake inhibitor; TCA, tricyclic antidepressant.

Pharmacologic Treatment of Anxiety

Choosing an Agent

- See p. 52 for a general discussion of diagnosis and treatment
- SSRIs and SNRIs are first-line agents for most of the disorders
- TCAs and MAOIs are effective but are typically associated with more side effects (*continued*)

TABLE 5-5 Selective Serotonin Reuptake Inhibitors

Agents (brand): citalopram (CIT; Celexa), escitalopram (ESC; Lexapro), fluoxetine (FLU; Prozac), fluvoxamine (FLV; Luvox; OCD only), paroxetine (PAR; Paxil), sertraline (SER; Zoloft)
Indications (FDA-approved indications in bold): MDD (all), GAD (ESC, SER), panic disorder (FLU, PAR, SER), OCD (FLU, FLV, PAR, SER), premenstrual dysphoric disorder (FLU, PAR, SER), social anxiety disorder (PAR, SER), bulimia
Contraindications: • Contraindicated with MAOI agents (washout ≥2 wks, ≥5 wks with fluoxetine) • Contraindicated with pimozide and thioridazine • Avoid other SSRIs, triptans, tryptophan, lithium, tramadol, linezolid, St. John's Wort, and fluconazole because of the risk of serotonin syndrome • Caution with NSAIDS (risk of GI bleeding) • Caution with diuretics (SIADH)
Adverse effects: **CNS:** mania; exacerbation of depression, suicidality, weakness, cognitive disturbances, somnolence, insomnia, seizures (rare) **GI:** nausea (improves later), xerostomia, anorexia or weight gain, diarrhea, increased LFTs (rare), GI bleed (rare), bruxism (rare)
Cardiovascular: arrhythmias (rare), decreased BP, dizziness **Metabolic:** sweating, rash or urticaria, bleeding (rare), hyponatremia, SIADH, increased blood glucose, gout, osteoporosis, galactorrhea **Urologic:** decreased libido, late ejaculation
Augmentation: bupropion, quetiapine, stimulants
Overdose: relatively safe
Withdrawal: symptoms include dizziness, lightheadedness, insomnia, fatigue, anxiety, agitation, nausea, headache
Metabolism: hepatic: 2D6: fluoxetine, paroxetine, sertraline, citalopram, escitalopram; 3A4/2C19: fluvoxamine
Pregnancy: category C

BP, blood pressure; CNS, central nervous system; FDA, Food and Drug Administration; GAD, generalized anxiety disorder; GI, gastrointestinal; LFT, liver function test; MAOI, monoamine oxidase inhibitor; MDD, major depressive disorder; NSAID, nonsteroidal antiinflammatory drug; OCD, obsessive–compulsive disorder; SIADH, syndrome of inappropriate antidiuretic hormone; SSRI, selective serotonin reuptake inhibitor.

(continued)

- MAOI use is supported by controlled trials in panic disorder, post-traumatic stress disorder and social anxiety disorder
- TCAs have no good evidence for use in patients with social anxiety disorder
- Benzodiazepine are efficacious, fast acting, and generally well tolerated but have abuse potential
- Studies have shown efficacy for buspirone, but results in clinical practice are less reliable *(continued)*

TABLE 5-6 Serotonin Norepinephrine Reuptake Inhibitors

Agents (brand): desvenlafaxine (DES; Pristiq), duloxetine (DUL; Cymbalta), venlafaxine (VEN; Effexor)

Indications (FDA-approved indications in bold): MDD (all), GAD (VEN), social phobia (VEN), panic disorder (VEN), diabetic neuropathy pain, fibromyalgia

Contraindications and interactions:
- Contraindicated with MAOI agents
- Use caution when using phenothiazine, TCAs, ciprofloxacin, ketoconazole,
- Use caution when using SSRIs, triptans, tryptophan, lithium, tramadol, linezolid, cyclobenzaprine, and St. John's Wort because these can lead to serotonin syndrome (see p. 41 for more information)
- Use caution in patients with glaucoma, seizure disorder
- Bulimia and alcohol dependence are relative contraindications

Adverse effects:
CNS: mania, agitation, depression exacerbation, suicidality (thoughts), asthenia or fatigue, dizziness, headache, insomnia or somnolence, tremor, blurred vision, seizures (rare)
GI: weight loss (rare gain), decreased appetite, nausea, constipation or diarrhea, xerostomia; bulimia and alcohol dependence are relative contraindications; increased LFTs

Cardiovascular: high BP (VEN: dose dependent), orthostatic decreased BP
Metabolic: increased blood glucose (rare), hyponatremia or SIADH (rare); increased sweating
Urologic: decreased libido, late ejaculation; urinary frequency or hesitation

Augmentation: mood stabilizers, atypical antipsychotics, Modafinil, benzodiazepines, gabapentin, lithium, buspirone, thyroid hormone; use caution with mirtazapine (two dual agents)

Overdose: relatively safe

Withdrawal: milder than with SSRIs (dizziness, lightheadedness, insomnia, fatigue, anxiety, agitation, nausea, headache, sensory disturbances)

Metabolism: hepatic: increased DUL levels with quinidine; decreased DUL levels with carbamazepine, phenobarbital, and rifampin

Pregnancy: category C

BP, blood pressure; CNS, central nervous system; FDA, Food and Drug Administration; GAD, generalized anxiety disorder; GI, gastrointestinal; LFT, liver function test; MAOI, monoamine oxidase inhibitor; MDD, major depressive disorder; SIADH, syndrome of inappropriate antidiuretic hormone; SSRI, selective serotonin reuptake inhibitor; TCA, tricyclic antidepressant.

(*continued*)

Dosages

- Start slow because patients with anxiety are very sensitive to somatic side effects
- Antidepressant doses used for depression are usually effective but in some cases it may be necessary to use higher doses

TABLE 5-7 Selective Serotonin Reuptake Inhibitors and Serotonin and Norepinephrine Reuptake Inhibitors

Medication and Route	Initial Dose (Dosing Range, mg/day)	Cost per Month (Average Dose)
Selective Serotonin Reuptake Inhibitors		
Citalopram (Celexa): 10-, 20-, and 40-mg tablets	10–20 (20–60)	$10 (20 mg/day) Celexa: $81
Escitalopram (Lexapro): 10- and 20-mg tablets 5-mg/5 mL solution	5–10 (10–20)	$84 (20 mg/day) No generic
Fluoxetine (Prozac): 10- and 20-mg tablets 20-mg/5 mL solution. 90-mg tablets (weekly)	10–20 (20–80)	$10 (20 mg/day) Prozac: $66 Weekly: $88 (30 mg)
Fluvoxamine (Luvox,-CR): 25-, 50-, and 100-mg tablets CR 100- and 150-mg tablets	25–50 (50–300)	$35 (100 mg/day) Luvox: $109 CR: $117
Paroxetine (Paxil, -CR): 10-, 20-, 30-, and 40-mg suspension CR 12.5, 25, 37.5 mg tablets	10–20 (20–60) (CR: 2.5–62.5)	$53 (30 mg/day), Paxil $90, CR $94
Sertraline (Zoloft): 25-, 50-, and 100- mg tablets	25–50 (50–200)	$13 (50 mg/day) Zoloft: $87
Serotonin and Norepinephrine Reuptake Inhibitors		
Desvenlafaxine (Pristiq): 50-mg tablets	50 (50–100)	$122 (50 mg/day)
Duloxetine (Cymbalta): 20-, 30-, and 60-mg tablets	20 (40–120)	$125 (60 mg/day)
Venlafaxine (Effexor, Effexor XR): regular: 25-, 37.5-, 50-, 75-, and 100-mg tablets XR: 150- and 300-mg tablets	75 (25–175) (TID dosing) XR: 25–50 (75–175)	$50 ($75 BID) Effexor: $135 XR: $107

BID, twice a day; TID, three times a day.

June 2008 average cost per month from online pharmacies.

(*continued*)

Monitoring

- Monitor adherence to prescribed treatment, particularly when prescribing medications with abuse potential

Changing and Augmenting Therapy

- Beta-blockers are sometimes used to reduce autonomic arousal in patients with panic attacks
- Beta-blockers are helpful to reduce performance anxiety, but not generalized anxiety or social phobia (*continued*)

TABLE 5-8 Tricyclic Antidepressants

Agents (brand): amitriptyline (Elavil), clomipramine (Anafranil), desipramine (Norpramin), doxepin (Sinequan), imipramine (Tofranil), nortriptyline (Pamelor), protriptyline (Vivactil), trimipramine (Surmontil)

Indications (FDA-approved indications in bold): MDD, enuresis (IMI), dysthymia, panic disorder, agoraphobia, bulimia, ADHD, diabetic neuropathy, urinary incontinence, disorders of ejaculation, pain, sleep disorders

Contraindications and interactions:
- Contraindicated with MAOIs (2-wk washout minimum)
- Contraindicated for acute post-MI
- Contraindicated in porphyria
- Use caution with QT-prolonging drugs such as haloperidol, quetiapine, risperidone, ziprasidone, venlafaxine and class I and III antiarrhythmics (beta-blockers, CCBs, clonidine, digitalis)
- Use caution with SSRIs, triptans tryptophan, lithium, tramadol, linezolid, St. John's Wort, (serotonin syndrome)
- Use caution with amphetamines (methylphenidate): increased cardiac side effects
- Use caution with anticoagulants (may increase plasma levels)
- Use caution with cimetidine

Adverse effects:
CNS: Suicidality, insomnia/nervousness, cognitive disturbances, delirium, paresthesias, tremor, blurred vision, rare seizures or tinnitus, increased risk of falls
GI: Constipation, ileus (rare), xerostomia (rare), hepatoxicity, weight gain
Cardiovascular: PR-prolongation, QTc prolongation, other ECG changes, arrhythmias, torsade de pointes (with risk of sudden death); all worse with overdoses
Metabolic: sweating, photosensitivity
Sexual: decreased libido, late ejaculation
Monitor: ECG, weight and BMI, glucose, lipid panel; if at risk for electrolyte disturbances, check K and Mg

Augmentation: lithium, lamotrigine, atypical antipsychotics, buspirone

Overdose: dangerous (arrhythmia); see p. 239

Withdrawal: rapid discontinuation may lead to sleep disturbance, GI distress, and mania

Metabolism: hepatic: 2D6 inhibitors (e.g., paroxetine) increase TCA levels

Pregnancy: category D

ADHD, attention-deficit hyperactivity disorder; BMI, body mass index; CCB, calcium channel blocker; ECG, electrocardiography; FDA, Food and Drug Administration; GI, gastrointestinal; IMI, imipramine; MAOI, monoamine oxidase inhibitor; MDD, major depressive disorder; MI, myocardial infarction; SSRI, selective serotonin reuptake inhibitor; TCA, tricyclic antidepressant.

(*continued*)

Maintenance

- The goal should be complete remission of symptoms
- Use of benzodiazepines should be time limited

Cessation

- Benzodiazepines must be tapered off slowly because of physiologic dependence (*continued*)

TABLE 5-9 Monoamine Oxidase Inhibitors

Agents: phenelzine (Nardil), tranylcypromine (Parnate), selegiline patch (EMSAM)

Indications (FDA-approved indications in bold): MDD, treatment-resistant depression, panic disorder, social anxiety disorder, bulimia

Contraindications and interactions:
- **Hypertensive crisis** with tyramine (or sympathomimetic-containing foods or drugs) with seizures, delirium, fever, collapse, coma, intracranial bleed; can block with phentolamine. Do not mix with other MAOIs; cocaine or other stimulants; OTC products with dextromethorphan, meperidine, or nasal decongestants; or appetite suppressants with sympathomimetic effects
- Avoid with SSRIs, tramadol, duloxetine, venlafaxine, buspirone, bupropion
- Do not use in the presence of recent cardiac event or CVA, headache, or liver disease
- Use caution with anesthetics and ziprasidone

Adverse effects:
CNS: insomnia, agitation, suicidality, sedation, dizziness, headache, fatigue, blurred vision, seizures (rare)
GI: constipation, xerostomia, hepatotoxicity (rare), weight gain, hypoglycemia in diabetics, increased LFTs

Cardiovascular: acute hypertension, orthostatic hypotension, sustained hypotension, arrhythmia
Sexual: decreased libido, late ejaculation

Augmentation: lithium, lamotrigine, atypical antipsychotics, buspirone

Overdose: may lead to agitation, hyperthermia, and hemodynamic instability

Withdrawal: minimal symptoms; as class, tapers over 2–3 weeks

Metabolism: hepatic CYP450 1A2

Pregnancy: category C

CNS, central nervous system; CVA, cerebrovascular accident; FDA, Food and Drug Administration; GI, gastrointestinal; LFT, liver function test; MAOI, monoamine oxidase inhibitor; MDD, major depressive disorder; OTC, over the counter; SSRI, selective serotonin reuptake inhibitor.

(continued)

Pregnancy

- All antidepressants are category C (some animal studies show adverse effects, but no controlled studies in humans are available) or D (there is evidence of risk to human fetuses, but the potential benefits may justify the risk)
- Benzodiazepines are category D (evidence of risk to human fetuses; potential benefits may justify the risk) or X (should not be used in pregnancy)
- Consider CBT, interpersonal therapy, supportive therapy, ECT, and hospitalization when medications are contraindicated

PHARMACOLOGIC TREATMENT OF BIPOLAR DISORDER

Choosing an Agent

- See p. 76 for a general discussion of diagnosis and treatment
- There is a significant risk of fetal malformation when using valproate and carbamazepine in women of childbearing age *(continued)*

TABLE 5-10 Tricyclic Antidepressants and Monoamine Oxidase Inhibitors

Medication and Formulations	Initial Dose (mg/day)	Dosing Range (mg/day)	Cost per Month (Average Dose)
Tricyclic Antidepressants			
Amitriptyline (Elavil): 10-, 25-, 50-,75-, 100-, and 150-mg tablets	25	50–300	$4 (75 mg/day)
Clomipramine (Anafranil): 25-, 50-, and 75-mg tablets	25	25–300	$35 (generic: 75 mg/day) $167 (brand: 75 mg/day)
Desipramine (Norpramin): 10-, 25-, 50-, 75-, 100-, and 150-mg tablets	25	25–300	$40 (100 mg/day)
Doxepin (Sinequan): 10-, 25-, 50-, 75-, 100-, and 150-mg tablets	25	25–300	$9 (generic: 75 mg/day) $28 (brand: 75 mg/day)
Imipramine (Tofranil): 10-, 25- and 5-mg tablets	25	50–300	$9 (50 mg/day) Tofranil: $173
Nortriptyline (Pamelor): 10-, 25-, 50-, and 75-mg tablets	25	75–150	$18 (generic: 150 mg/day) $622 (brand: 150 mg/day)
Protriptyline (Vivactil): 5-, and 10-mg tablets	10–15	15–60	$155 (30 mg/day)
Trimipramine (Surmontil): 25-, 50-, and 100-mg tablets	20–30	50–300	$97 (100 mg/day)
Monoamine Oxidase Inhibitors			
Phenelzine (Nardil): 15 mg tablets	30	50 mg	$60 (75 mg/day)
Tranylcypromine (Parnate): 10-mg tablets	30	40–120	$100 (30 mg/day)
Selegiline patch (EMSAM): 6-,9-, and 12-mg patches	6–12 q24 hr	6–12 q24 hr	$460 (6 mg/day)

TABLE 5-11 Alternative and Adjunctive Agents for the Treatment of Depression

Generic (Brand) and Formulations	Initial Dose (mg/day)	Dosing Range (Total mg/day)	Cost per Month (Average Dose)	Clinical Considerations
Bupropion: Wellbutrin-SR, Wellbutrin-XL, Zyban) 75-, and 100-mg tablets SR: 100- and 150-mg tablets XL: 150-, and 300-mg tablets	25–50 (TID dosing) SR: 50–100 (BID dosing) XL: 150 (QD dosing)	150–450 (TID dosing) SR: 100–400 (BID dosing) XL: 150-450 (QD dosing)	$86 (300 mg) $116 (300 mg as brand-SR) $125 (300 mg as brand-XL)	• Often used as adjunctive medication with SSRIs and SNRIs • Fewer sexual side effects than with SSRIs and SNRIs • Lowers seizure threshold
Buspirone (BuSpar as an adjunct): 5-, 10-, 15-, and 30-mg tablets	15	15–60	$23 (20 mg)	• Often used as an adjunctive medication for anxiety and depression
Mirtazapine (Remeron): 15-, 30-, and 45-mg tablets	15	15–45	$46 (generic 30 mg) $93 (brand 30 mg)	• Used as an adjunctive medication or as second-line agent, particularly for patients with insomnia
Nefazodone (Serzone): 50-, 100-, 150-, 200-, and 250-mg tablets	100	100–600	$50 (150 mg)	• Limited use because of cases of hepatotoxicity (need to follow LFTs in patients)
Olanzapine + fluoxetine (ODC, Symbyax): 6 + 25-mg, 6 + 50-mg, 12 + 5-mg, 12 + 25-mg, 12 + 50-mg tablets	6 + 25	6 + 25–12 + 50	$300 (6 + 25 mg)	• Recently released agent • See side effects for olanzapine

BID, twice a day; LFT, liver function test; QD, every day; SNRI, serotonin and norepinephrine reuptake inhibitor; SSRI, selective serotonin reuptake inhibitor; TID, three times a day.

TABLE 5-12 Agents Used to Treat Anxiety Disorders

Drug	Initial Dose (Dosing Range, mg/day)	Advantages	Disadvantages
Selective Serotonin Reuptake Inhibitors *Please refer to Table 5-5 for class specific information*			
Citalopram (Celexa) **Escitalopram** (Lexapro) **Fluoxetine** (Prozac) **Fluvoxamine** (Luvox) **Paroxetine** (Paxil) **Paroxetine CR** (Paxil CR) **Sertraline** (Zoloft)	10–20 (20–60) 10 (10–30) 10 (10–80) 50 (50–300) 10 (10–50) 12.5 (12.5–50) 25 (25–100)	• Low abuse risk • May dose once daily • Low interaction risk • Low toxicity with overdose	• May increase anxiety initially • Common sexual and GI dysfunction • Delayed onset of action
Mixed Serotonin and Norepinephrine Reuptake Inhibitors *Please refer to Table 5-6 for class specific information*			
Duloxetine (Cymbalta) **Venlafaxine XR** (Effexor XR)	40 (40–120) (may use divided dosing) 37.5 (75–375)	• Fast acting • Well tolerated	• May increase anxiety, agitation, or initially • Common sexual and GI dysfunction • Delayed onset of action • Venlafaxine may cause elevated BP
Benzodiazepines (Selected) *Please refer to Table 5-30 for class specific information*			
Alprazolam (Xanax) **Clonazepam** (Klonopin) **Diazepam** (Valium) **Lorazepam** (Ativan)	0.25–0.5 (2–10) (TID dosing) 0.5 (1–5) (BID dosing) 5 (5–40) (BID, TID, or QID dosing) 1–2 (3–16) (TID or QID dosing)	• Fast acting • Well tolerated • Low cost	• High abuse liability • Risk of withdrawal syndrome • Dissociation, sedation • Ataxia • Requires multiple doses per day if short half life
Tricyclic Antidepressants (Selected) *Please refer to Table 5-8 for class specific information*			
Amitriptyline (Elavil) **Clomipramine** (Anafranil) **Imipramine** (Tofranil)	10–25 (50–300) 12.5–25 (100–250) 10–25 (50–300)	• Low cost • Once-daily dosing • Very well studied and long used	• Clomipramine is also an SNRI • Not well tolerated • Anticholinergic effects • Sedating

(*continued*)

TABLE 5-12 Agents Used to Treat Anxiety Disorders (*continued*)

Drug	Initial Dose (Dosing Range, mg/day)	Advantages	Disadvantages
		• Option when modern agents fail	• Cardiac depressants • Toxic; lethal on overdose
Monoamine Oxidase Inhibitors *Please refer to Table 5-9 for class specific information*			
Phenelzine (Nardil) **Selegiline** (Eldepryl) **Selegiline patch** (EMSAM) **Tranylcypromine** (Parnate)	15 (60–90) (daily or BID) 5–10 (10–20) 6 (12) 10–20 (20–60) (BID dosing)	• Efficacious in treatment-refractory cases	• Dietary restrictions to avoid hypertensive crises with sympathomimetics (e.g., tyramine, NeoSynephrine) • Many drug interactions (e.g., SSRIs, methylphenidate) • Toxic; lethal on overdose
Atypical Antipsychotics *Please refer to Table 5-20 for class specific information*			
Aripiprazole (Abilify) **Olanzapine** (Zyprexa) **Risperidone** (Risperdal and Consta) **Quetiapine** (Seroquel) **Ziprasidone** (Geodon)	2 (2–30 2.5 (2.5–30) 0.25–0.5 (0.5–6) 12.5 (25–400) (daily or divided dosing) 40 (40–160)	• Aggressively marketed • Good studies for other indications	• Not well studied for treatment of anxiety • Risk of metabolic syndrome • Some EPS risk (especially akathisia, atypical NMS; TD with risperidone)
Anticonvulsants *Please refer to Table 5-13 for class specific information*			
Carbamazepine (Tegretol) **Gabapentin** (Neurontin) **Levetiracetam** (Keppra)	250 (400–1000) 500 (1000–2000) 500 (2000–3000)	• Aggressively marketed	• In most cases, not proven effective to treat anxiety; benefits are often exaggerated

(continued)

TABLE 5-12 Agents Used to Treat Anxiety Disorders (*continued*)

Drug	Initial Dose (Dosing Range, mg/day)	Advantages	Disadvantages
Oxcarbazepine (Trileptal) **Valproate** (Depakote)	250 (600–1800) 250–500 (1000–2000)		• May produce dependence and risk seizures on stopping • Tremor • Alopecia • Sedating • Weight gain • Highly teratogenic (carbamazepine, valproate) • Valproate can masculinize with PCOS • Drug interactions (carbamazepine induces metabolism of many agents; valproate increases lamotrigine) • Levetiracetam has some evidence of anxiolytic effects (off-label use) • Gabapentin and oxcarbazepine are off-label use for psychiatry
Adrenergic Agents			
Clonidine (anti-α_2) (Catapres) **Prazosin (anti-α_1)** (Minipress) **Propranolol (anti-β)** (Inderal)	0.1 (0.1–2.4) 1 (1–15) 20 (40–60)		• Off-label use in psychiatry • May lower heart rate and BP
Antihistamines			
Diphenhydramine (Benadryl) **Hydroxyzine** (Vistaril)	12.5–25 (25–50) 25–50 (75–400)	• Relatively safe • Long used	• Sedating • Anticholinergic effects

(*continued*)

TABLE 5-12 Agents Used to Treat Anxiety Disorders (*continued*)

Drug	Initial Dose (Dosing Range, mg/day)	Advantages	Disadvantages
Miscellaneous			
Bupropion SR (Wellbutrin SR) **Bupropion XL** (Wellbutrin XL) **Buspirone** (BuSpar) **Trazodone** (Desyrel)	100 (300–400) (BID dosing) 150 (300–450) 5 (15–60) (BID or TID dosing) 25 (50–200)	• Buspirone and trazodone lack the addictive properties of benzodazepines • Bupropion (Zyban) is also indicated for smoking cessation	• Bupropion: marketed at suboptimal doses; mild stimulant (risks agitation, insomnia); may induce seizures • Buspirone is not highly effective for treating anxiety • Trazodone is not very effective; side effects include priapism and sedation

BID, twice a day; BP, blood pressure; EPS, extrapyramidal side effects; GI, gastrointestinal; NMS, neuromalignant syndrome; PCOS, polycystic ovarian syndrome; QID, four times a day; SNRI, serotonin and norepinephrine reuptake inhibitor; SSRI, selective serotonin reuptake inhibitor; TD, tardive dyskinesia; TID, three times a day.

Adapted from Iosifescu D, Pollack M: An approach to the anxious patient: symptoms of anxiety, fear, avoidance, or increased arousal. In Stern TA (ed). *The Ten-Minute Guide to Psychiatric Diagnosis and Treatment.* New York, NY: Professional Publishing; 2005:205.

(*continued*)

- If an agent works for acute mania, it can be continued for maintenance
- Antipsychotics used in the acute manic phase should be discontinued upon stabilization unless they are being used to treat psychosis

Dosages

- Medications should be titrated to effectiveness with drug levels checked on a schedule

Monitoring

- Valproate and lithium require careful monitoring of levels, particularly at the outset of treatment
- Renal and hepatic function should be monitored regularly

Changing and Augmenting Therapy

- Augmentation for depressive symptoms is often necessary, although there is a risk of inducing mania with the addition of antidepressants

Pregnancy

- Lithium, valproate, and carbamazepine are category D (evidence of risk to human fetuses; potential benefits may justify the risk)
- Valproate is teratogenic and associated with neural tube defects

TABLE 5-13 Mood-Stabilizing Agents

Agents	Initial Dose (Dosing Range), mg)	Therapeutic Consideration
Standard Agents		
Lithium carbonate and citrate (Lithobid): 150-, 300-, and 600-mg tablets	300–600 (600–2400) (divided doses)	• Before use, check creatinine, BUN, TSH, electrolytes, ECG (age >50 years), body weight • Adjust for acute trough levels of 0.8–1.2 mEq/L with maintenance levels of 0.50–0.75 mEq/L • Two or three times a year, recheck Li, electrolytes, TSH, CBC, ECG, creatinine; also check dose-changes, adding drugs, or suspected toxicity (may include creatinine clearance and urine osmolarity)
Valproate (Depakote, ER): 125-, 250-, and 500-mg tablets and oral suspension	250–500 (1200–1500)	• Hepatic failure risk factors: infants, multiple anticonvulsants, higher doses, dementia • Follow CBC, especially in the early months • Dose using ≤10–20 mg/kg/day with a goal blood level of 45–125 μg/mL
Carbamazepine (Tegretol): 100-, 200-, and 400-mg tablets oral suspension	200–600 (400–1200) (divided doses)	• Before use, check Na, CBC, BUN, creatinine, LFTs, TSH, weight • Follow CBC and Na every 2–4 wks for 8 wk and then every 3–6 mo • Follow BUN, creatinine, LFTs, and TSH every 6–12 mo
Lamotrigine (Lamictal): 2-, 5-, 25-, 100-, 150-, and 200-mg tablets	12.5–25 (200–300)	• Must be titrated slowly because of concern for Stevens-Johnson syndrome • Avoid new foods and medicines • Watch for any rash
Non–FDA-approved Agents		
Topiramate (Topamax): 15-, 25-, 100-, and 200-mg tablets	25–50 (50–300) (adjunctive)	• Check baseline and occasional bicarbonate (non–anion gap metabolic acidosis) • Watch for sedation, weight loss, confusion, kidney stones
Gabapentin (Neurontin): 100-, 300-, 400-, 600-, and 800-mg tablets	300–600 (800–2400) (divided doses)	• Watch for dizziness, drowsiness, peripheral edema, toxicity in renal impairment

BUN, blood urea nitrogen; CBC, complete blood count; ECG, electrocardiography; FDA, Food and Drug Administration; LFT, liver function test; Li, lithium carbonate; TSH, thyroid-stimulating hormone.

TABLE 5-14 Lithium Carbonate (Li+)

Indications (FDA-approved indications in bold): bipolar disorder maintenance, manic episode to augment antidepressants, aggressive behavior, schizoaffective disorders (not well studied), suicidal behaviors, headache

Contraindications and interactions:
- Decreased lithium levels: acetazolamide, bicarbonate, sodium polystyrene (Kayexalate)
- Increased lithium levels: diuretics, ACE inhibitors, NSAIDs, COX-2 inhibitors, indomethacin, sartans, metronidazole
- Use caution with antipsychotics (risk of delirium with confusion, EPS, fever)
- Use caution with SSRIs, triptans, tryptophan, tramadol, linezolid, St. John's Wort (serotonin syndrome with delirium–see page 41 for more information)
- Use caution with verapamil (neurotoxicity, bradycardia)
- Use caution with α-methyldopa, carbamazepine, phenytoin (toxicity)
- Avoid during ECT (stop ≥1 wk before and restart several days after ECT)

Adverse effects:
CNS: Sedation, cognitive disturbances, tremors, hypertonicity, choreoathetotic movements, hyperactive DTRs, EPS, acute dystonia, ataxia and cerebellar disorders, headache, seizures (rare), pseudotumor cerebri, or encephalopathic delirium (weakness, lethargy, fever, tremor, confusion, EPS, leukocytosis, elevated serum enzymes, BUN, blood glucose)
GI: weight gain, anorexia, xerostomia, nausea, vomiting, diarrhea
Cardiovascular: T-wave flattening, conduction abnormalities, arrhythmias, bradycardia
Dermatologic: alopecia, acne, folliculitis, worsens psoriasis
Urologic: polyuria, polydipsia, nephrogenic diabetes insipidus, interstitial nephritis or nephrotic syndrome (rare), chronic renal failure, fluid or electrolyte abnormalities, sexual dysfunction

Augmentation: valproate, lamotrigine, other anticonvulsants, antipsychotics, antidepressants (poor long-term outcomes)

Overdose: see Lithium toxicity (p. 44)

Withdrawal: risk of early recurrence of depression or mania (within months), depression in early pregnancy after rapidly stopping lithium (taper over ≥1 mo)

Metabolism: renal GFR 10–50 mL/min; decrease dose 50%–75% if GFR <10 mL/min or by 25%–50% with prior renal or nephritic illness; avoid salt and water depletion or concurrent use of thiazide diuretics or NSAIDs

Pregnancy: category D (10x increase to one in 1500 of Ebstein's anomaly), although relatively safe compared with other mood stabilizers

ACE, angiotensin-convertin enzyme; BUN, blood urea nitrogen; CNS, central nervous system; COX, cyclooxygenase; DTR, deep tendon reflexes; ECT, electroconvulsive therapy; EPS, extrapyramidal side effects; FDA, Food and Drug Administration; GI, gastrointestinal; GFR, glomerular filtration rate; NSAID, nonsteroidal antiinflammatory drug; SSRI, selective serotonin reuptake inhibitor.

TABLE 5-15 Valproate (Depakote, VPA)

Indications (FDA-approved indications in bold): seizure disorder (partial-complex, absence), mania, bipolar disorder prophylaxis, migraines, neuropathic pain as adjunct to antidepressants, and augmentation of antipsychotics
Contraindications and interactions: • May increase tissue levels of lamotrigine by two to three times • Use caution with carbamazepine, phenytoin, rifampin (lower levels) • Expect higher serum drug level with salicylates, chlorpromazine, fluoxetine, fluvoxamine, topiramate, cimetidine, erythromycin, ibuprofen • Safe with lithium and antipsychotics
Adverse effects: **CNS:** Sedation, tremors, dizziness, ataxia, weakness, headache, cognitive disturbance **GI:** nausea, vomiting, diarrhea, abdominal pain, constipation, dyspepsia, weight gain, pancreatitis (rare), hepatotoxicity (rare) **Dermatologic:** rash, alopecia (rare) **Hematologic:** dose-related thrombocytopenia **Metabolic:** PCOS, hyperinsulinemia, lipid dysregulation
Augmentation: lamotrigine, other anticonvulsants, antipsychotics, antidepressants (poor long-term outcomes)
Overdose: most cases are benign, although toxicity (multiple CNS symptoms, including coma, confusion, somnolence) may occur in overdose or with high valproate level caused by inappropriate dosing or poor metabolism
Withdrawal: avoid abrupt discontinuation (increased risk of status epilepticus)
Metabolism: hepatic
Monitoring: serum levels, LFTs, coagulation, CBC, body weight, BMI, glucose, cholesterol, triglycerides
Pregnancy: category D: associated with multiple birth defects, including three to five in 100 chance of spina bifida (poorly countered with folate)

BMI, body mass index; CBC, complete blood count; CNS, central nervous system; FDA, Food and Drug Administration; LFT, liver function test; PCOS, polycystic ovarian syndrome.

PHARMACOLOGIC TREATMENT OF PSYCHOSIS

Choosing an Agent

- See p. 92 for general discussion of diagnosis and treatment
- Most antipsychotics are similarly efficacious in schizophrenia for the long term but may differ in the short term (mania, acute psychosis). Agents differ widely differ in potency, adverse effects, routes of administration, cost, marketing levels, and popularity
- **Older, first-generation or typical neuroleptics:** chlorpromazine, fluphenazine, haloperidol (*continued*)

TABLE 5-16 Carbamazepine (Tegretol)

Indications (FDA-approved indications in bold): epilepsy (partial, generalized tonic-clonic), trigeminal neuralgia, acute or mixed mania and mixed state, bipolar disorder prophylaxis, used empirically as an adjunct to antipsychotics (but lowers drug levels; some increased risk of Stevens-Johnson syndrome, especially in Asians with the HLA-B-1502 allele)
Contraindications and interactions: • Avoid with MAOI ≥2 wks (risk of delirium) • Avoid with risks factors for blood dyscrasias and osteoporosis • Avoid with known porphyria, hepatic impairment, glaucoma • Fluvoxamine > fluoxetine increases levels of carbamazepine • Use caution with acetaminophen, clomipramine, benzodiazepines, haloperidol, anticonvulsants, anticoagulants, oral contraceptives • Lithium rarely may increase the risk of CNS effects • Safe with antipsychotics, valproate, lamotrigine
Adverse effects: **CNS:** Sedation, tremors, dizziness, ataxia, weakness, headache, cognitive disturbance, ataxia, blurred vision **GI:** nausea, vomiting, constipation or diarrhea, weight gain **Cardiovascular:** arrhythmia (rare) **Dermatologic:** rash; Stevens-Johnson syndrome (rare), diaphoresis **Endocrinologic:** SIADH (rare) **Metabolic:** aplastic anemia or agranulocytosis (rare) leukopenia, SIADH (rare but more common with oxcarbazepine) **Urologic:** urinary retention
Augmentation: valproate, lamotrigine, other anticonvulsants, antipsychotics, antidepressants (poor long-term outcomes)
Overdose: symptoms may include dizziness, sedation, seizures, tachycardia
Withdrawal: avoid abrupt discontinuation (status epilepticus)
Metabolism: hepatic via CYP450 3A4
Monitoring: CBC, LFTs, creatinine, TSH, Na
Pregnancy: category D: strongly associated with multiple birth defects, including one in 100 chance of spina bifida

CBC, complete blood count; CNS, central nervous system; FDA, Food and Drug Administration; LFT, liver function test; MAOI, monoamine oxidase inhibitor; SIADH, syndrome of inappropriate antidiuretic hormone; TSH, thyroid-stimulating hormone.

(*continued*)

- Extrapyramidal side effects (EPS) (rigidity, bradykinesia, tremor, akathisia, NMS) are common
- There is about a 5% to 7% per year risk of tardive dyskinesia (TD); the risk is higher in elderly individuals
- Increased prolactin, galactorrhea, amenorrhea may occur
- Weight gain (*continued*)

TABLE 5-17 Lamotrigine (Lamictal)

Indications (FDA-approved indications in bold): maintenance treatment of bipolar I disorder, partial seizures in adults and children older than age 2 years, bipolar depression, bipolar mania (adjunctive), psychosis and schizophrenia (adjunctive)
Contraindications and interactions: • Valproate increases plasma concentrations, requiring half the dosing or less of lamotrigine • Oral contraceptives may lower levels • Safe with lithium and antipsychotics
Adverse effects: rare multiorgan failure associated with Stevens-Johnson syndrome or drug hypersensitivity syndrome **CNS:** sedation, dizziness **GI:** nausea, vomiting, diarrhea, abdominal pain, constipation, dyspepsia, **Dermatologic:** rash may be benign (10%) or serious; monitor closely **Hematologic:** blood dyscrasias (rare)
Augmentation: valproate, other anticonvulsants, antipsychotics
Overdose: symptoms include ataxia, nystagmus, seizures, and coma
Withdrawal: avoid abrupt discontinuation because the patient is at risk for seizure recurrence and recurrence of bipolar depression
Metabolism: hepatic with renal excretion
Monitoring: monitor closely when starting medication, specifically looking for rash; if any widespread or pruritic rash occurs (or other laboratory abnormalities), discontinue (as well as valproate if in conjunction) and monitor closely with full laboratory tests; the patient may require hospitalization
Pregnancy: category D: associated with multiple birth defects, including a three in five of 100 chance of spina bifida (poorly countered with folate)

FDA, Food and Drug Administration; CNS, central nervous system; GI, gastrointestinal.

(continued)

- **Modern, second-generation, and atypical antipsychotics:**
  - Decreased risk of Most acute EPS
  - Decreased risk of TD
  - **Risperidone:** extensive clinical experience; patent ending and cost are already relatively low; available in disintegrating tablet, liquid and depot formulations; the risk of EPS (especially akathisia and perhaps TD) is higher than with other modern agents and is dose dependent; moderate weight gain and clinically significant prolactin elevation are possible side effects
  - **Olanzapine:** wide clinical experience; varied routes of administration; may have superior adherence in maintenance; weight gain and risk for metabolic syndrome are high; costly
  - **Quetiapine:** low EPS-incidence, even at higher doses; need high doses for antipsychotic effects; wide range of doses and utility; causes sedation

(continued)

TABLE 5-18 Typical Antipsychotics (Neuroleptics)
Agents: chlorpromazine (Thorazine), fluphenazine (Prolixin), haloperidol (Haldol, and depot), molindone (Moban), perphenazine (Trilafon), pimozide (Orap), thioridazine (Mellaril), trifluoperazine (Stelazine)
Indications (FDA-approved indications in bold): schizophrenia, psychosis, Tourette's syndrome (haloperidol, pimozide), dementia, agitation, delirium, bipolar disorder, severe behavioral problems
Contraindications and interactions: • Caution: CV disease, narrow-angle glaucoma, hepatic disease, myasthenia, Parkinson's disease, epilepsy
Adverse effects: **CNS:** sedation or agitation, blurred vision, EPS (parkinsonian bradykinesia with variable tremor, acute dystonia, akathisia, TD, NMS) **GI:** constipation, weight gain, xerostomia, esophageal dysmotility, ileus **Cardiovascular:** arrhythmias, sudden death, QT prolongation, orthostasis **Dermatologic:** hyperpigmentation, photosensitivity **Metabolic:** blood dyscrasias (monitor CBC), increased prolactin, (amenorrhea, galactorrhea), pigmentary retinopathy (rare) **Urologic:** urinary retention (rare), priapism
Augmentation: lithium, lamotrigine, atypical antipsychotics, buspirone
Overdose: symptoms can include delirium, coma, respiratory depression, and seizures; important to monitor medically
Withdrawal: abrupt discontinuation may lead to rebound psychosis
Metabolism: hepatic CYP450 system
Pregnancy: category C

CBC, complete blood count; CV, cardiovascular; EPS, extrapyramidal side effects; FDA, Food and Drug Administration; NMS, neuromalignant syndrome; TD, tardive dyskinesia.

(continued)

hypotension and a moderate risk of weight gain; twice-daily dosing is needed

- **Aripiprazole:** long elimination half-life; low risk of weight gain or EPS (but not well tolerated by psychotic Parkinson patients); lack of cardiac effects; long half-time; risk of agitation
- **Ziprasidone:** low risk of weight gain, injectable; twice-daily dosing, potential QT prolongation, risk of agitation
- **Paliperidone (9-OH-risperidone):** once-daily dosing; new and costly; little advantage over generic risperidone
- **Clozapine:** effective in otherwise poorly responsive patients; potential lethality secondary to pancytopenia; requires white blood cell monitoring; weight gain is a possible side effect; may require months to assess effects adequately (*continued*)

TABLE 5-19 Typical Antipsychotic Agents

Medication and Route	Initial Dose (Dosing Range, mg/day)	Cost per Month (Average Dose,)
Chlorpromazine (Thorazine): 10-, 15-, 25-, 50-, 100-, 150-, and 200-mg tablets' liquid	10–50 (30–800)	$10 (200 mg/day)
Fluphenazine (Prolixin): oral: 1-, 2.5-, 5-, and 10-mg tablets IM: decanoate 25 mg/5 mL	5–10 (oral: 1–40; IM: 12.5–37.5 every 2–3 wk)	$25 (20 mg/day) $60 (25 mg/day IM for 2 wks)
Haloperidol (Haldol, and depot): 0.5-, 1-, 2-, 5-, 10-, and 20-mg tablets	2–10 (oral: 1–20; IM: 100–200)	$13 (20 mg/day)
Molindone (Moban): 5-, 10-, 25-, and 50-mg tablets	10–20 (5–225)	not available
Perphenazine (Trilafon): 2-, 4-, 8-, and 16-mg tablets	4–16 (12–64)	$42 (16 mg/day)
Pimozide (Orap): 1- and 2-mg tablets	1–2 (1–10)	$80 (4 mg/day)
Thioridazine (Mellaril): 10-, 15-, 25-, 50-, 100-, 150-, and 200-mg tablets	20–100 (20–800)	$25 (200 mg/day)
Trifluoperazine (Stelazine): 1-, 2-, 5-, and 10-mg tablets	20 (15–20)	$40 (15 mg/day)

IM, intramuscular.

(*continued*)

Dosing

- Usually increased to average therapeutic dose as quickly as the patient can tolerate, with the exception of clozapine, which must be titrated more slowly given concerns for pancytopenia
- Calming effect usually immediate; delusions and hallucinations require 1 to 8 weeks; other effects are variable

Monitoring

- Patients taking clozapine require regular monitoring of WBC and absolute neutrophil count

Changing and Augmenting Therapy

- Avoid the impulse to change medication or dose quickly; cross-titrate agents gradually; poor data are available regarding most combinations with other APDs or other classes (*continued*)

TABLE 5-20 Atypical (Second-Generation) Antipsychotics

Agents: aripiprazole (ARI; Abilify) clozapine (CLZ; Clozaril), olanzapine (OLZ; Zyprexa; IM: Zydis), paliperidone (PAL; Invega), risperidone (RIS; Risperdal), quetiapine (QUE; Seroquel), ziprasidone (ZIP; Geodon)
Indications (FDA-approved indications in bold): schizophrenia (all), psychosis (all), depression (ARI, SER), mania (ARI), bipolar disorder prophylaxis, agitation in any form, impulse-control disorders, possibly in some treatment-resistant anxiety
Contraindications and interactions: • Caution: CV disease, narrow-angle glaucoma, hepatic disease, myasthenia, Parkinson's disease, epilepsy
Adverse effects: **CNS:** sedation or agitation, EPS (parkinsonism, acute dystonia, akathisia, TD, NMS), blurred vision **Gastrointestinal:** constipation, weight gain, xerostomia, esophageal dysmotility **Dermatologic:** hyperpigmentation, photosensitivity **Cardiovascular:** variable QT prolongation (ziprasidone), arrhythmias, orthostatic hypotension, sudden death **Hematologic:** blood dyscrasias
Augmentation: lithium, lamotrigine, typical antipsychotics, buspirone, SSRIs, SNRIs
Overdose: signs and symptoms may include delirium, coma, respiratory depression, and seizures; it is important to monitor medically
Withdrawal: abrupt discontinuation may lead to rebound psychosis
Metabolism: hepatic CYP 450 system
Pregnancy: category C

CV, cardiovascular; EPS, extrapyramidal side effects; FDA, Food and Drug Administration; NMS, neuromalignant syndrome; SNRI, serotonin and norepinephrine reuptake inhibitor; SSRI, selective serotonin reuptake inhibitor; TD, tardive dyskinesia.

(*continued*)

Maintenance

- Review periodically (≥3 months) to adjust dose to current clinical needs vs. tolerability
- Monitor weight and body mass index (BMI), hyperglycemia, dyslipidemia, and blood pressure

Cessation

- Abrupt discontinuation may lead to rebound psychosis

Pregnancy

- Typical and atypical antipsychotics seem to be associated with an increased risk of neonatal complications; however, their use during pregnancy is indicated when risk to the fetus from exposure to this medication is outweighed by the risks of untreated psychiatric illness in the mother (*continued*)

TABLE 5-21 Modern (Atypical) Antipsychotics

Medication (Trade Name) and Formulations	Initial Dose (Dosing Range, mg/day)	Cost per Month (Average Dose)
Aripiprazole (Abilify): 2-, 5-, 10-, 15-, 20-, and 30-mgtablets and 1-mg/mL liquid	10–50 (2–30)	$393 (15 mg/day)
Clozapine (Clozaril): 25-, 50-, 100-, and 200-mg tablets	12.5–25 (25–800)	Generic: $303 (300 mg/day) Brand: $492 (300 mg/day)
Olanzapine (Zyprexa, IM: Zydis): 2.5-, 5-, 7.5-, 10-, and 15-mg tablets Zydis: 5-, 10-, 15-, and 20-mg tablets	5–10 (2.5–30)	Oral: $347 (10 mg/day) Zydis: $405 (10 mg/day)
Paliperidone (Invega): 3-, 6-, 9-, and 12-mg tablets	3–6 (6–12)	$351 (6 mg/day)
Risperidone (Risperdal, Consta, Risperdal M-disintegrating tabs): 0.25-, 0.5-, 2-, 3-, and 4-mg tablets Consta: 12.5-, 25-, 37.5-, and 50-mg IM	2–4 (4–10) 25–50 mg IM 2–6 mg PO QD	Oral: $375 (4 mg/day) M: $444 (4 mg/day) Consta: $440 (25 mg/day q2wk)
Quetiapine (Seroquel): 25-, 100-, 200-, and 300-mg tablets	25–50 (50–800)	$230 (200 mg/day)
Ziprasidone (Geodon): 20-, 40-, 60-, and 80-mg tablets	20–40 (40–160)	$331 (40 mg/day)

IM, intramuscular; QD, every day.
June 2008 average cost from online pharmacies.

(*continued*)

- All antipsychotics are category C (some animal studies show adverse effects, but no controlled studies in humans are available) or D (there is evidence of risk to human fetuses, but the potential benefits may justify the risk)

Geriatrics

- Increased mortality (cerebrovascular accident [CVA], myocardial infarction [MI]) with dementia-related-psychosis has been associated with older and newer agents

Pediatrics

- Few antipsychotics are approved for patients younger than age 12 years; the benefits often nonspecific or unclear; there are severe risks of weight gain and metabolic syndrome

PHARMACOLOGIC TREATMENT OF DEMENTIA

Principles

- See p. 58 for general discussion of diagnosis and treatment
- Consider depression, anxiety, and medical disorders, as either causes or comorbidities
- Begin treatment early to slow the progression and to delay nursing-home placement
- Increase dose slowly every 2–4 wks
- If medications are changed, slowly cross-titrate
- Evaluate treatment results over months

TABLE 5-22 Treatments for Dementia

Drug	Uses	Forms (Dosing)	Cost per Month (Average Dose)	Adverse Effects
Cholinesterase Inhibitors (Acetylcholinesterase Inhibitors)				
Donepezil (Aricept, Memac)	All stages	5- and 10-mg tablets (5–10 mg/day slow increase)	$170 (5 mg/day)	Nausea, vomiting, anorexia, diarrhea, syncope, seizures (rare)
Galantamine (Razadyne, ER)	Mild to moderate	4-, 8-, and 12-mg tablets; 4-mg/mL liquid (1–24 mg/day slow increase)	$18 (16 mg/day)	Nausea, vomiting, anorexia (should be taken with food), diarrhea, syncope, seizures (rare)
Rivastigmine (Exelon, Patch)	Mild-moderate	1.5-, 3-, and 4.5-mg tablets; 2-mg/mL liquid (3–6 mg/day slow increase)	$173 (3 mg/day)	Nausea, vomiting, anorexia, diarrhea
Tacrine (Cognex)	Mild-moderate	10-, 20-, 30-, and 40-mg tablets (40–1600 mg/day increased over 1 month)	$350 (40 mg/day)	Possible liver damage (follow LFTs), nausea, vomiting
N-Methyl-D-Aspartate Receptor Antagonist				
Memantine (Namenda)	Moderate-severe	5- and 10-mg tablets; 2-mg/mL liquid (5–40 mg/day slow increase)	$166 (20 mg/day)	Headache, confusion, dizziness, constipation; can be added to ACh inhibitors safely

Ach, acetylcholinesterase; LFT, liver function test.

TABLE 5-23 Cholinesterase Inhibitors

Agents (brand): donepezil (Aricept, Memac), galantamine (Razadyne, -ER) rivastigmine (Exelon, -Patch) tacrine (Cognex)

Indications (FDA-approved indications in bold): Alzheimer's disease, mild to moderate dementia, memory disorders, mild cognitive impairment

Contraindications and interactions:
- Caution with anesthetics/surgery, levodopa, cholinomimetics, anticholinergics
- Use caution with beta-blockers (bradycardia) and with heart block
- Use caution: peptic ulcer, asthma, liver disease, renal impairment

Adverse Effects:
CNS: insomnia, dizziness, fatigue, seizures (rare)
GI: nausea, diarrhea, vomiting, anorexia
Cardiovascular: rare syncope
Drug specific:
- **Tacrine:** liver toxicity
- **Donepezil:** bradycardia, syncope, mild GI side effects
- **Rivastigmine:** significant GI side effects, anorexia, weight loss

Overdose: symptoms consistent with anticholinergic overdose

Withdrawal: significant worsening of dementia may occur with discontinuation and may continue until restarting or using another agent

Metabolism: hepatic CYP450 mediated metabolism

Pregnancy: category C

CNS, central nervous system; FDA, Food and Drug Administration; GI, gastrointestinal.

TABLE 5-24 N-Methyl D-Aspartate Receptor Antagonists

Agent (brand): memantine (Namenda)

Indications: moderate to severe Alzheimer-type dementia and in other memory disorders, mild cognitive impairment

Contraindications and interactions:
- Use caution with amantadine, ketamine, dextromethorphan
- Safe to combine with cholinesterase inhibitors
- Safe with antidepressants, valproate, carbamazepine and oxcarbazepine and sometimes combined with antipsychotics despite their risk to increase mortality in such patients

Adverse effects:
CNS: sedation, dizziness, confusion, headache, seizures (rare)
GI: constipation

Withdrawal: significant worsening of dementia can occur with discontinuation and may continue until restarting or using another agent

Metabolism: hepatic

Pregnancy: category C

CNS, central nervous system; GI, gastrointestinal.

Pharmacologic Treatment of Attention-Deficit Hyperactivity Disorder

- See p. 115 for general discussion of diagnosis and treatment
- Stimulants are prescribed in limited amounts to limit risks of diversion, abuse, or overdose
- Avoid in patients with current substance abuse; use caution in patients with a history of substance abuse
- Monitor for agitation, irritability, and suicidality, especially early and with dose changes
- **Atomoxetine** is less effective but is not a controlled substance; it has also been associated with rare but severe liver injury
- **Cardiovascular events**, including sudden death in adults (CVA, MI) and juveniles with structural abnormalities or other serious heart problems have been reported

TABLE 5-25 Stimulants

Agent (brand): mixed amphetamines (Adderall, -XR), dextroamphetamine (Dexedrine), methylphenidate (Ritalin, -LA, Concerta; Daytrana patch), lisdexamfetamine (Vyvanse)
Indications (FDA-approved in bold): ADHD, narcolepsy (long acting preferred), treatment-resistant or residual depression (adjunctive)
Contraindications and interactions: • Use caution: risk of dependence or abuse, tolerance, psychosis, anxiety, new tics or worsening of Tourette syndrome • Use caution with hypertension, hyperthyroidism, epilepsy, glaucoma, cardiac abnormalities • Use caution with BP medications, clonidine, anticoagulants, steroids • Use caution with anticonvulsants, TCAs, mood stabilizers • Avoid all MAOIs
Adverse effects: **CNS:** insomnia, agitation, headache, tics, tremor, psychosis, seizures, NMS (rare) **GI:** anorexia, nausea, abdominal pain, diarrhea; weight loss, retarded growth in children **Cardiovascular:** tachycardia, hypertension, arrhythmias, sudden death
Hematologic: leucopenia or anemia (rare)
Overdose: symptoms may include vomiting, agitation, tremors, hyperreflexia, cardiac arrhythmias, hypertension, confusion, hallucinations, flushing, headache, hyperpyrexia, tachycardia, palpitations
Monitoring: BP, height and weight, growth (children), CBC with special attention to platelets, LFTs
Withdrawal: recurrence of depressive symptoms, agitation (most often seen in patients abusing medication)
Metabolism: hepatic
Pregnancy: category C

ADHD, attention-deficit hyperactivity disorder; BP, blood pressure; CBC, complete blood count; FDA, Food and Drug Administration; LFT, liver function test; MAOI, monoamine oxidase inhibitor; NMS, neuromalignant syndrome; TCA, tricyclic antidepressant.

TABLE 5-26 Treatments for Attention-Deficit Hyperactivity Disorder

Stimulants

Generic (Brand)	Forms	Dose	Indications	Cost (Dose)	Adverse Effects
Mixed amphetamines (Adderall, -XR)	5-, 7.5-, 10-, 12.5-, 15- ,20- and 30-mg tablets	RR: 5–40 mg/day XR: 5–60 mg/day	ADHD (any age), narcolepsy	Generic: $82 (10 mg/day) Brand: $120 (10 mg/day)	Class risks: anorexia, weight loss, induction of mania, hypomania, mixed states in bipolar disorder, worsening or induction of psychosis, new tics or worsening of Tourette syndrome, hypertension, cardiac dysfunction; use with caution with known bipolar disorder, psychosis, epilepsy, hypertension, cardiac disease
Dextroamphetamine (Dexedrine)	5-, 10-, and 15-mg tablets	5–60 mg/day	ADHD, narcolepsy	$21 (20 mg/day)	
Methylphenidate (Ritalin, -LA, Concerta; Daytrana patch)	5-, 10-, and 20-mg tablets Patch: 10-, 15-, 20-, and 30-mg	SR: 20 mg/day LA: 20 mg/day Concerta: 18 mg/day 10–60 mg/day	ADHD	Generic: $21 (20 mg/day) Ritalin: $33 (20 mg/day) Ritalin-SR: $55 (20 mg/day) Ritalin-LA: $97 (20 mg/day) Concerta $107 (18 mg/day) Ritalin-patch: $150 (15 mg/day)	

(continued)

TABLE 5-26 Treatments for Attention-Deficit Hyperactivity Disorder (*continued*)

Generic (Brand)	Forms	Dose	Indications	Cost (Dose)	Adverse Effects
Stimulants					
Lisdexamfetamine (Vyvanse)	30-, 50-, and 70-mg tablets	30–70 mg/day		$123 (30 mg/day)	
Nonstimulants					
Atomoxetine (Strattera)	10-, 18-, 25-, 40-, and 60-mg tablets	40–100 mg/day	ADHD	$126 (10 mg/day)	Tachycardia, hypertension, urinary retention, constipation, liver toxicity
Modafinil (Provigil)	100- and 200-mg tablets	200 mg/day	Narcolepsy, other sleep disorders, shift-work, OSA	$213 (200 mg/day)	Headache, anxiety, insomnia, xerostomia, diarrhea

ADHD, attention-deficit hyperactivity disorder; **OSA**, obstructive sleep apnea.

Pharmacologic Treatment of Substance Use Disorders

- See p. 102 for general discussion of diagnosis and treatment

TABLE 5-27 Food and Drug Administration–Indicated Pharmacologic Treatments for Alcohol Dependence

Medication and Route	Actions	Therapeutics	Limitations, Contraindications, and Side Effects
Disulfiram Antabuse: 125–500 mg/day PO	**Aversion to drinking** • Inhibits aldehyde dehydrogenase, blocking the metabolism of acetaldehyde, a toxic intermediate of alcohol metabolism • Accumulation of acetaldehyde causes uncomfortable autonomic symptoms (nausea, vomiting, diarrhea, flushing)	• Makes alcohol psychologically unavailable because of the aversive "disulfiram reaction" • Useful in well-motivated patients with close monitoring (e.g., parents or professionals being monitored for sobriety and at risk of losing their children or job) • Requires daily medication adherence and careful dose titration • May be used episodically (e.g., during times of high risk)	• Contraindicated in patients with severe cardiac and coronary disease (causes an acute increase in BP) • Idiosyncratic hepatic failure in one of 50,000 patients (monitor LFTs) • Avoid other sources of alcohol (e.g., mouthwash, hand sanitizer) • Binge drinking is potentially fatal

(continued)

TABLE 5-27 Food and Drug Administration–Indicated Pharmacologic Treatments for Alcohol Dependence (*continued*)

Medication and Route	Actions	Therapeutics	Limitations, Contraindications, and Side Effects
Naltrexone: • PO: ReVia 25–100 mg/day • IM: Vivitrol 380 mg Q4wk	• Opioid antagonist at the μ-opioid receptor • Reduces positive reinforcement associated with alcohol use by decreasing the associated central dopamine release	• Promotes abstinence by reducing "reward craving" • May reduce the intensity and frequency of cravings to drink • Decreases the chances of a lapse progressing to full relapse • As effective as behavioral interventions in achieving abstinence after detoxification • IM for noncompliant patients (need wallet card)	• Contraindicated in patients who need opioid agonist medications • Nausea and headache are common, sometimes transient side effects • Hepatotoxicity (reversible and dose dependent; use with caution in patients with liver disease)
Acamprosate Campral: 666 mg PO TID (titrate from 333 mg TID for 1 week to avoid initial GI side effects)	• Glutamate receptor modulator • Decreases symptoms (dysphoria, anxiety, irritability, restlessness) during the early period of abstinence	• Promotes abstinence by reducing early abstinence syndrome • In patients who have completed detoxification, helps to increase sober time during follow-up • Useful in patients with liver disease • To be used as monotherapy (no benefit as an add-on to naltrexone or disulfiram)	• Frequency of diarrhea at initiation can be lessened by slower titration • Contraindicated in patients with poor renal fnction

BP, blood pressure; GI, gastrointestinal; IM, intramuscular; LFT, liver function test; TID, three times a day.

TABLE 5-28 Food and Drug Administration–Indicated Pharmacologic Treatments for Nicotine Dependence

Medication and Route	Actions	Therapeutics	Limitations, Contraindications, and Side Effects
Nicotine replacement therapy: • **Patch:** 7–28 mg • **Lozenge:** 2–4 mg • **Nasal spray:** 2 puffs per nostril **Inhaler:** puff frequently for 20 minutes	• Alternative routes of nicotine administration • Nicotine is not carcinogenic (other components of cigarettes are carcinogenic)	• All have similar efficacy at alleviating withdrawal symptoms and reducing smoking • Plan to completely replace usual nicotine intake (1 mg per cigarette; 20 per pack) or to decrease by <25% initially and then wean off • Patch delivers a steady level, reducing cravings and withdrawal and may be combined with other methods for breakthrough cravings • Nasal spray delivers the highest dose	• May cause local irritation • Recommend carrying surgical or duct tape and spare patches because they may come off • Recommend removing patch before sleep because of increased nightmares or restlessness
Bupropion (Zyban): 150 mg PO BID (titrate from 150 mg QD for 3 days)	• Antidepressant that acts as a weak norepinephrine and dopamine reuptake inhibitor and an antagonist of nicotinic acetylcholine receptors • Unclear which specific mechanism(s) are responsible for clinical efficacy of bupropion as an antidepressant and smoking cessation agent	• Same efficacy as NRTs at alleviating withdrawal symptoms and reducing smoking • Begin 1 week before quit date • May combine with NRT • Improves quit success rate • May reduce weight gain associated with quitting smoking	• Contraindicated in patients with predisposition to seizures • May cause insomnia and "jitters" • Carefully monitor patients with bipolar disorder for emergence of mania

(*continued*)

TABLE 5-28 Food and Drug Administration–Indicated Pharmacologic Treatments for Nicotine Dependence (*continued*)

Medication and Route	Actions	Therapeutics	Limitations, Contraindications, and Side Effects
Varenicline tartrate (Chantix): 1 mg PO BID (titrate up from 0.5 mg/day for 3 days and then 0.5 mg BID for 4 days)	• Partial agonist at nicotinic cholinergic receptors • Mildly activates receptor but competitively blocks exogenous nicotine from binding to receptors	• Treat for 12–24 weeks beginning one week before quit date	• Withdrawal if discontinued abruptly • Recent warnings about neuropsychiatric side effects

BID, twice a day; NRT, nicotine replacement therapy; PO, oral; QD, every day.

TABLE 5-29 Food and Drug Administration–Indicated Pharmacological Treatment for Opioid Dependence

Medication and Route	Actions	Therapeutics	Limitations, Contraindications, and Side Effects
Methadone (Dolophine, Methadose): 20–120 mg/day	• Opioid replacement therapy • Long-acting, μ-opioid receptor agonist that minimizes euphoria but prevents opiate withdrawal, blocks the effects of illicit opiates, and reduces opiate craving	• Safe and effective for maintenance of abstinence • Used in the outpatient setting to facilitate patient participation in behavioral therapies • Prescribed at certified opioid treatment programs	• Many drug–drug interactions • Contraindicated with severe respiratory disease • May induce "opiate apathy," depressed mood, weight gain, constipation, sedation, respiratory depression • QTc prolongation

(*continued*)

TABLE 5-29 Food and Drug Administration–Indicated Pharmacological Treatment for Opioid Dependence (*continued*)

Medication and Route	Actions	Therapeutics	Limitations, Contraindications, and Side Effects
Buprenorphine (Subutex, Suboxone [buprenorphine + naloxone]**)**: 4–32 mg/day SL	• Opioid replacement therapy • Partial agonist at μ-opioid receptors; prevents opiate withdrawal, blocks the effects of illicit opiates, and reduces opiate craving • Suboxone combines buprenorphine (absorbed SL) with naloxone (not absorbed SL), a short-acting opioid antagonist • Naloxone is active if injected IV, thereby preventing diversion of buprenorphine for misuse	• Improved safety and tolerability compared with full opioid agonists • First-line treatment when available • Buprenorphine may be delivered in routine, office-based practices • Opioid-dependent individuals do not experience euphoria with buprenorphine	• Contraindicated with benzodiazepine misuse • May induce withdrawal if given shortly after opioid use • Monitor LFTs more closely for patients with HCV or other liver diseases
Naltrexone: 25–50 mg/day PO only	• Long-acting synthetic opioid receptor antagonist that blocks the effects of opioid agonists at their receptors • No addictive potential • Intended to help the patient "unlearn" habits by blocking desired opiate effects	• For use 7–10 days after detoxification (otherwise could precipitate withdrawal symptoms); usually initiated at transition from inpatient detoxification to an outpatient setting • Limited by low rates of patient adherence and treatment retention	• Risk of opioid overdose either because of attempt to overcome receptor blockade with high doses of opioids or because of opioid use after discontinuation when opioid receptors have become sensitized by medication • Hepatoxicity (monitor LFTs)

HCV, hepatitis C virus; IV, intravenous; LFT, liver function test; SL, sublingual.

SEDATIVE–HYPNOTICS

TABLE 5-30 Sedative–Hypnotics

Generic (Brand)	Dose (Ativan-eq)	Half-Life (hr)	Onset	Active Metabolites (Half-Life, hr)	Administration	Metabolism	Dose (mg/day)
Benzodiazepines							
Alprazolam (Xanax, XR)	0.5	6–27	Fast to intermediate	No (6–27)	PO	Hepatic	0.75–5.00
Chlordiazepoxide (Librium, Mitran)	10	8–28	Intermediate	Yes (3–200)	PO	Hepatic	15–100
Clonazepam (Klonopin)	0.5	18–50	Slow	No (19–50)	PO	Hepatic	0.5–4.0
Clorazepate (Tranxene)	7.5	30–200	Fast	Yes (3–200)	PO	Hepatic	15–60
Diazepam (Valium)	5	20–50	Fast	Yes (3–200)	PO, IV	Hepatic	4–40
Flurazepam (Dalmane)	15	40–114	Fast	Yes (36–120)	PO	Hepatic	15–30
Lorazepam (Ativan)	1.0 (comparator)	10–20	Intermediate	No (13–16)	PO, IV, IM	Hepatic and renal	1–10
Midazolam (Versed)	2	1–4	Fast	No	IV, IM	—	—

Benzodiazepines							
Oxazepam (Serax)	15	5–15	Slow to intermediate	No	PO	Hepatic and renal	30–120
Temazepam (Restoril)		3.5–18.5	Fast	No	PO	Hepatic and renal	15–30
Triazolam (Halcion)		1.5–5.5	Fast	No	PO	Hepatic	0.125–0.5
Other Hypnotics							
Eszopiclone[a] (Lunesta)		3–6	Fast	No	PO	Hepatic	1–3
Ramelteon[b] (Rozerem)		1–3	Fast	No	PO	Hepatic	8–16
Zaleplon[a] (Sonata)		1	Fast	Yes	PO	Hepatic	5–20
Zolpidem[a] (Ambien, -CR, Stilnox)		1.5–4.5	Fast	No	PO	Hepatic	5–10 CR: 6.25–12.5

[a]Benzodiazepine receptor agonists. May afford less tolerance and dependence; similar impairments of memory or performance; and lack the anxiolytic, anticonvulsant, and muscle-relaxant properties of benzodiazepines. Use is restricted to 35 days.

[b]Melatonin-receptor agonist; approved for adults with difficulty initiating sleep.

IM, intramuscular; IV, intravenous; PO, oral.

TABLE 5-31 Other Sedating Drugs

Generic (Brand)	Action	Dose (mg/day)	Side Effects and Contraindications
Diphenhydramine (Benadryl)	Antihistamine	25–300 PO or IM (divided)	CNS depressant May be clinically dangerous with emphysema, COPD, glaucoma, BPH
Benztropine (Cogentin)	Anticholinergic	0.5–2	Use caution in patients with glaucoma, tachycardia, BPH
Hydroxyzine (Vistaril, Atarax)	Antihistamine	50–100 PO or IM	Dry mouth, drowsiness Avoid long-term use in patients with anxiety
Promethazine (Phenergan)	Phenothiazine	12.5–50	High risk of typical EPS May produce fatal respiratory depression Use caution in patients with glaucoma, ulcer, obstrutions, hepatic disorders, marrow dysfunction or depressants, epilepsy
Melatonin (unbranded)	Hormone	0.5–10	Use caution in patients with bleeding and those using anticoagulants, NSAIDs, antiplatelet or antidiabetic agents

COPD, chronic obstructive pulmonary disease; EPS, extrapyramidal side effects; BPH, benign prostatic hypertrophy; IM, intramuscular; NSAID, nonsteroidal antiinflammatory drug; PO, oral.

TABLE 5-32 Herbal Medications Used in Psychiatry

Agent	Indications	Dose (mg/day)	Adverse Risks	Efficacy
St. John's Wort	Mild to moderate depression	300–1800 (divided)	Serotonin syndrome with SSRIs; may induce CYP3A4 9 and lower OCPs, cyclosporin, digoxin, Indinavir, Irinotecan, warfarin levels); mania, phototoxicity, dry mouth, dizziness, constipation anxiety, fatigue, headache, sexual dysfunction	Poor evidence in severe MDD One RCT in moderate MDD

(continued)

TABLE 5-32 Herbal Medications Used in Psychiatry (*continued*)

Agent	Indications	Dose (mg/day)	Adverse Risks	Efficacy
SAMe	Depression; may augment antidepressants	400–1600	May increase mania or anxiety in bipolar disorder, mild insomnia, decreased appetite, constipation, nausea, dry mouth; sweating, dizziness	May be effective if given IV; RCTs about PO administration are ambiguous; sometimes used to augment SSRIs or SNRIs
Folate	Depression; may augment antidepressants; may help in mild dementia	.4 (RDA age 19 years and older)	High doses may provoke vitamin B12 deficiency; may interact with methotrexate; may increase seizure risk at high doses and with anticonvulsants; may cause allergic reactions	Decreased folate levels are linked with decreased response to antidepressant treatment
Omega-3 fatty acids	Depression > mania in bipolar disorder	1000–2000 (EPA + DHA)	GI distress, fishy taste, may induce mania, may increase bleeding with anticoagulants	May be effective in bipolar depression for long-term use (off-label use); may augment antidepressants

DHA, docosahexaenoic acid; EPA, eicosapentaenoic acid; GI, gastrointestinal; IV, intravenous; MDD, major depressive disorder; OCP, oral contraceptive pills; PO, oral; RCT, randomized, controlled trial; RDA, recommended daily allowance; SAMe, S-adenosyl methionine; SNRI, serotonin and norepinephrine reuptake inhibitor; SSRI, selective serotonin reuptake inhibitor.

General Guidelines for the Management of Non-Emergent Side Effects

- Educate patients about common, serious, and transient side effects before initiating a new medication
- Begin with the lowest effective dose and gradually titrate upward ("start low; go slow")
- Reassure and wait when side effects are likely to abate with ongoing therapy.
- Consider adjunctive agents rather than switching to another agent, which may delay the therapeutic response

- Inform patients that some psychiatric symptoms mirror common side effects of psychiatric medication (e.g., sexual dysfunction associated with both SSRIs and major depressive disorder)

ANTIDEPRESSANTS

Sexual Dysfunction (SSRIs, SNRIs > TCAs, MAOIs)

- Spectrum of symptoms: decreased libido, decreased arousal, anorgasmia, erectile dysfunction, ejaculation latency
- Clinically more commonly reported than package inserts indicate (≤20% for most SSRIs; up to 50% with fluoxetine)
- Underreported unless specifically screened for
- Not likely to resolve without intervention
- Idiosyncratic class effect, in that different SSRIs and SNRIs may cause varying degrees of sexual effects
- **Management:**
  - Decrease the dose (poorly studied, but a reasonable first step; risks of diminishing antidepressant efficacy)
  - Switch to another SSRI (but no definitive comparison studies exist)
  - Switch to bupropion, nefazodone, or mirtazapine (there is some randomized, controlled trial support for less association with sexual symptoms)
  - Add a second drug as adjunct:
    - Sildenafil: 50–100 mg (trials show improved erection, orgasm, and ejaculation in men)
    - Bupropion: 100–300 mg/day (RCTs show improved libido in women)
    - Buspirone: 15–60 mg/day (conflicting RCT data)
    - Cyproheptadine, amantadine, yohimbine, stimulants (inconclusive anecdotal data)
  - Drug holiday (not well studied or supported)

Gastrointestinal Effects (TCAs, SSRIs, SNRIs)

- Common early; transient effects seen with many psychotropics
- Appear within days of drug initiation or dose increase but often resolve within 2 weeks without intervention
- Nausea, vomiting, and dyspepsia:
  - Common effect of all SSRIs and SNRIs (reported by 25% to 40% of patients)
  - More common with sertraline, fluvoxamine, and duloxetine
  - Less associated with enteric-coated, controlled-release formulations
  - Minimize by starting at a low dose and taking after meals
  - Treatment of nausea and vomiting: ondansetron, metoclopramide, trimethobenzamide
  - Treatment of dyspepsia: reduce alcohol, caffeine, and fatty foods; over-the-counter antacids (Milk of Magnesia, Maalox, Mylanta, Pepto-Bismol, Tums), H2 blockers

- Diarrhea and constipation:
  - Paroxetine is the SSRI that is most often associated with constipation
  - Treatment of constipation: increase dietary fluid and fiber intake; fiber supplements (psyllium), stool surfactants (docusate sodium), laxatives (Milk of Magnesia, lactulose, bisacodyl, senna, polyethylene glycol)
  - Treatment of diarrhea: switch to paroxetine; loperamide, diphenoxylate or atropine

Sedating and Activating Central Nervous System Effects (SSRIs, SNRIs, Mirtazapine, Trazodone)

- Spectrum of possible effects ranging from sedation to "activation" (anxiety, insomnia, jitteriness)
- Idiosyncratic effects in that a given drug might be sedating for one patient and activating for another
- Paroxetine, mirtazapine, and trazodone tend to be sedating; fluoxetine is activating
- Anxiety and jitteriness are often early, transient effects that improve within 2 weeks and can be prevented by starting at low doses or managed with benzodiazepines
- Insomnia may improve with reducing caffeine, eliminating daytime naps, practicing good sleep hygiene, and providing hypnotics or low-dose trazodone

Weight Gain (TCAs = MAOIs, Mirtazapine > SSRIs, SNRIs, Bupropion)

- Likely mediated by H1 and 5HT2C receptors
- Paroxetine is associated with the greatest weight gain among the SSRIs
- Unlike other antidepressants, bupropion causes appetite suppression more often than appetite enhancement
- Treatment: dietary modification, exercise programs, switch to bupropion, add topiramate (associated with weight loss)
- Also see Antipsychotics and Mood Stabilizers

Alopecia (SSRIs)

- Tends to be diffuse, nonscarring alopecia that may be localized or generalized and commonly affecting the scalp
- May appear immediately after drug initiation or months later
- Treatment: discontinue offending drug (typically reversible)

Anticholinergic Effects (TCAs > SSRIs, Mirtazapine)

- See Antipsychotics

Bleeding and Bruising (SSRIs)

- Anecdotal reports of higher incidence of easy bruising, petechiae, purpura, epistaxis, hematomas
- Retrospective data suggest an increased need for transfusions during surgery

- Case-control data suggest risk of non-gastrointestinal (GI) bleeding may be higher if the patient is taking nonsteroidal antiinflammatory drugs or anticoagulants (but no increased risk of GI bleeding)
- Mechanism may be related to the effects of serotonin on platelet aggregation

Mood Stabilizers

Cognitive Impairment (Lithium, Valproate, Topiramate)

- Mood stabilizers may induce subjective impairment in concentration, memory, creativity, spontaneity, or language (speech, word finding)
- Difficult to distinguish cognitive impairment from fatigue, sedation, even mild depression, hypomania, or Li-induced hypothyroidism
- Cognitive effects also are seen in placebo -arms of trials and among euthymic bipolar disorder patients, and imply illness as well as treatments causes
- Management:
  - Rule out associated causes of cognitive impairment (Li-induced hypothyroidism, residual depression)
  - Reduce Li dose or switch to controlled-release formation (Lithobid); reduce other suspected agents

Tremor (Lithium, Valproate, Lamotrigine)

- Most common is a rapid, dose-related, benign, postural tremor (8–12 Hz), especially of the hands; exacerbated by fine motor control or social stress
- Over longer-term therapy, features of tremor can become Parkinsonian
- Severe or sudden worsening suggests lithium toxicity (see p. 44 for more information)
- Management:
  - Wait (nontoxic tremor often improves spontaneously) or decrease the dose
  - Eliminate all caffeinated beverages
  - Switch to slow-release Li preparation (Lithobid)
  - Prescribe a beta-adrenergic antagonist (propanolol 30–220 mg/day, divided)
  - Prescribe other adjuncts (primidone, gabapentin)

Gastrointestinal Effects (Lithium, Valproate, Lamotrigine)

- Diarrhea, nausea, and vomiting are common with mood stabilizers
- Management:
  - Dose with meals
  - Reduce lithium dosing to one to two times/day
  - Switch to an enteric-coated or controlled-release preparation (e.g., slow-release Li [Lithobid], divalproex sodium [Depakote and ER])
  - H2-blockers may counter nausea with valproate

Dermatologic Effects

- About 10% of patients develop dermatologic reactions to psychiatric medications

- The usual reaction is a benign, self-limited, erythematous, maculopapular rash occurring early in treatment
- Acne and psoriasis are exacerbated or caused by Li; omega-3 fatty acids may counter psoriasis
- Alopecia is rarely associated with lithium and valproate; multivitamins fortified with zinc or selenium may help
- Rash (lamotrigine, carbamazepine lithium, valproate):
  - Rashes associated with mood stabilizers require discontinuation more than other psychotropics
  - The likelihood of rash may be reduced with slower dose titration (especially with lamotrigine)
  - Advise patients to avoid new medications, foods, and products during the first 3 months of using lamotrigine
  - Benign rashes: nonconfluent, nontender, maculopapular, and peaking within days and improving within 2 weeks; systemic signs are absent
    - Management:
      - Reduce the drug dose or postpone any scheduled increase (especially if lamotrigine)
      - Warn the patient to stop the drug if the rash worsens; monitor closely
      - Prescribe an antihistamine and topical steroids for pruritus
  - Nonbenign rashes: Confluent, widespread, purpuric, tender, vesicles or bullae; seen on the upper trunk, neck, mouth, lips, or eyes; systemic signs include fever, malaise, high WBC, liver function tests, /blood urea nitrogen, creatinine
    - Management: drug discontinuation and medical management

Weight Gain (Lithium, Valproate, Carbamazepine)

- Monitor weight and BMI before and during treatment; screen for prediabetes, diabetes, dyslipidemia, and hypertension
- Variably associated with increased appetite
- Lithium-induced weight gain may be higher in women than men
- Management:
  - Exercise and dietary modification (restrict carbohydrates; may counter insulin-like lithium effect)
  - Rule out lithium-induced subclinical hypothyroidism as a contributor to weight gain
  - Switch to lamotrigine (weight neutral) or add topiramate to other mood stabilizers (for weight loss, not efficacy)

Polyuria and Polydipsia (Lithium)

- Often appear transient and resolve with ongoing use but persist in 25% on long-term Li maintenance
- When severe, may represent nephrogenic diabetes insipidus (lithium decreases renal sensitivity to antidiuretic hormone)
- Management:
  - Maintain the lowest effective trough lithium level
  - Switch to once-daily dosing if tolerated

- Diuretics (amiloride, HCTZ or triamterene): decrease lithium dose by 50% and follow levels closely; amiloride spares K+

ANTIPSYCHOTICS

EPS (Extrapyramidal side effects)

(High-potency neuroleptics > Low-potency older neuroleptics > Modern antipsychotics at moderate doses)

- Related to D2 receptor blockade in nigrostriatal pathway, balanced by excitatory cholinergic activity
- Acute dystonia:
  - Definition: intermittent but sustained spasms of the head and neck muscles leading to involuntary movements (especially on days 2 to 10 as bradykinesia evolves; few are immediate)
  - Torticollis or retrocollis of the neck muscles, oculogyric crisis (eyes turn upward), laryngospasm (tongue or throat muscles contract leading to respiratory distress if severe), opisthotonos (patient arches forward)
  - Risk factors: youth, muscular males, high-potency neuroleptics
  - Not observed with clozapine
  - Dystonias of laryngeal or pharyngeal muscles are a rare cause of sudden death and require intubation if severe
  - Management: anticholinergics (benztropine 1–2 mg orally [PO], intramuscularly [IM], or intravenously [IV]; diphenhydramine 25–50 mg PO, IM, or IV)
- Akathisia:
  - Definition: sensation of motor restlessness associated with a strong desire to move the lower extremities, usually occurring within 1 month, but can appear anytime
  - Signs and symptoms: pacing, agitation, inability to keep the legs still or remain still in a chair, shifting weight from foot to foot
  - May begin as subjective feeling of inner restlessness before increased motor activity becomes apparent
  - Dose-related effect
  - Subjectively very unpleasant and may drive patients to non-adherence and even suicide
  - Often mistaken for agitation, leading clinicians to increase the antipsychotic dose and thereby worsen symptoms
  - Management:
    - Reduce antipsychotic dose
    - Benzodiazepines (lorazepam 0.5 mg three times a day)
    - Beta-blockers (propanolol 20 mg four times a day)
- Parkinsonism:
  - Signs and symptoms: rigidity, bradykinesia, tremor, mask facies, shuffling and festinating gait usually occurring within 5 to 30 days
  - Initial signs may be a diminished arm swing or decreased facial expressiveness
  - Difficult to distinguish certain parkinsonian symptoms from negative symptoms of schizophrenia or depressive symptoms

- Dose-related effect
- Risk factors: elderly, prior episode of EPS, high-potency typicals
- Management:
  - Reduce antipsychotic dose
  - Anticholinergics (benztropine 1–2 mg twice a day), amantadine 100–200 mg twice a day
- **TD (Typicals > Atypicals > Clozapine)**
  - Definition: movement disorder involving involuntary movements of mouth, tongue, and upper extremities usually appearing after chronic antipsychotic treatment (>6 months)
    - The cause may be related to increased dopamine (DA) receptor sensitivity in the basal ganglia (response to chronic DA-R blockade)
    - Perioral movements are most common (chewing; lip licking; smacking or puckering; tongue protrusion; grimacing; blinking), but choreoathetoid movements of the fingers or toes and writhing movements of the trunk are also observed
  - Differential diagnoses: Huntington's disease, Wilson's disease, Sydenham's chorea, hyperthyroidism, hypoparathyroidism, tardive Tourette's
  - Risk of developing TD on typical antipsychotics is around 5% per year of exposure (for at least the first 4 years of treatment)
  - Risk factors: elderly, female, treatment duration of longer than 6 months, comorbid mood disorder, diabetes, prior parkinsonism
  - Remission is most likely if the onset was recent or before age 40 years
  - Clozapine is less likely to cause TD, and many clinical reports suggest that it can suppress TD
  - Abnormal involuntary movement scale (AIMS) assessment is used to regularly examine patients for TD
  - Management:
    - Reevaluate the need for continued antipsychotic treatment with the patient and family
    - Reduce the antipsychotic to the lowest effective dose
    - Switch to an atypical (or to a different atypical)
    - Trial of clozapine
    - Vitamin E: 800–1200 IU/day as an adjunct (there have been mixed results in small randomized trials)

Metabolic Effects (Typical and Atypical Antipsychotics)

- Routinely monitor weight, BMI, fasting lipid panel, fasting glucose, waist circumference (at umbilicus), and blood pressure
- Identify risk factors: personal or family history of HTN, dyslipidemia, obesity, diabetes, cardiovascular disease
- All are treated with standard lifestyle changes and medical management when necessary
- **Weight gain** (low-potency typicals > high-potency typicals > clozapine, olanzapine > other atypicals)
  - Highest-risk atypicals: clozapine (75% of patients; average, 10- to 25-lb weight gain), olanzapine

- Lowest-risk atypicals: ziprasidone, aripiprazole
- Lowest-risk typical: molindone (may actually cause weight loss)
- The mechanism unclear but may be mediated by H1 and 5HT2C receptors
- Diabetes mellitus, type 2 (clozapine, olanzapine > other atypicals > typicals)
  - Range of manifestations from borderline glucose elevation to severe diabetic ketoacidosis
  - Highest risk: clozapine, olanzapine (but associated with all atypicals and typicals)
  - Mechanism may relate to insulin overutilization (resulting from weight gain) or development of insulin resistance
- Dyslipidemia
  - Most common type is hypertriglyceridemia
  - Mechanism is unknown

Sialorrhea (Clozapine > Typicals > Atypicals)

- Particularly common with clozapine (~80% of patients) but has been observed with all antipsychotics
- Increase in secretory saliva flow (under parasympathetic control) or impaired swallowing ("pool and drool")
- Etiology: drug-induced parkinsonism (bradykinesia lowers rate of swallowing), α2 blockade, M4 receptor agonism, excessive sedation
- May increase the risk of choking, aspiration pneumonia, salivary gland swelling or inflammation
- Management:
  - Speech and swallow evaluation to rule out surgically amenable conditions
  - Decrease dose (although no clear relationship between clozapine dose and drooling severity)
  - Sugarless gum
  - Systemic anticholinergics: atropine, benztropine, trihexyphenidyl, amitriptyline, glycopyrrolate
  - Local anticholinergics: sublingual or intranasal ipratropium spray
  - Central α2 agonists: clonidine patch, guanfacine
  - Botulinum toxin injections into parotid gland for refractory cases

Hyperprolactinemia (Typicals, Risperidone > Other Atypicals)

- Related to D2 receptor blockade in tuberoinfundibular tract (where DA typically inhibits prolactin release)
- Signs and symptoms: galactorrhea, oligomenorrhea or amenorrhea, gynecomastia, sexual dysfunction
- Management: decrease dose or switch agents

Orthostatic Hypotension (Low-Potency Typicals > High-Potency Typicals > Atypicals)

- May result in fainting or falls, especially in elderly or patients with impaired balance
- Tolerance to this effect may develop gradually

- Management:
  - Switch to a higher-potency agent
  - Instruct the patient to sit with the feet on the floor before standing up slowly and to sit or lie down when feeling faint
  - Nonpharmacologic interventions: stockings, volume expansion with intravenous fluids or increased oral fluid intake
  - Pressors (last resort)

Anticholinergic Effects (Low-Potency Typicals > High-Potency Typicals > Atypicals)

- Signs and symptoms: use the mnemonics "blind as a bat" (blurred vision, mydriasis), "dry as a bone" (xerostomia), "mad as a hatter" (delirium), "stuck as a pig" (constipation, urinary retention)
- Tolerance often develops to these effects with ongoing antipsychotic treatment
- Urinary retention may be complicated by urinary tract infection, renal damage (especially in elderly, benign prostatic hyperplasia, outflow abnormalities)
- Dry mouth may cause bad breath, stomatitis, or dental caries; treat with sugarless gum or hard candy and rinse the mouth often
- Blurred vision may improve with cholinergic agonists (pilocarpine 1% eye drops, bethanechol)

Somatic Therapies

Electroconvulsive Therapy

- **Description:**
  - Controlled induction of seizure activity using electrical stimulation in the brain while the patient is under anesthesia
  - Most established somatic therapy; first-line treatment for refractory depression
  - Greatest demonstrated efficacy of all treatments for major depressive disorder
- **Indications and target populations**
- **Relative indications:**
  - Rapid antidepressant effect required
    - Acute suicidality
    - Food refusal and nutritional compromise
    - Patient preference
  - History of prior good response to ECT
  - Refractory to antidepressant medication
- **Contraindications:**
  - No absolute contraindications
  - Relative contraindications:
    - Cardiovascular disease (because of transient increases in heart rate and blood pressure from ECT treatment) *(continued)*

TABLE 5-33 Indications for Electroconvulsive Therapy

Main Indications	Other Indications
Major depression	Dysthymia
Bipolar depression	Psychosis NOS
Psychotic depression	Parkinson's disease
Acute mania or mixed state	NMS
Schizophrenia	Delirium
Catatonia	Status epilepticus

NMS, neuroleptic malignant syndrome; NOS, not otherwise specified.

(continued)

- HTN, coronary artery disease, unstable aneurysm, arrhythmia, pacemaker
- Aortic stenosis (critical stenosis ≤0.9 cm^2)
- Cerebral risk factors
  - Increased intracranial pressure: space-occupying lesion, hydrocephalus
  - Infarct or hemorrhage, dementia, aneurysm, arteriovenous malformation, seizure disorder
- Pregnancy (because of the risk of anesthesia)
- Any contraindication to specific anesthetics: use of propofol or succinylcholine

- **Complications:**
  - Cognitive
    - Acute confusion or delirium
    - Short-term memory loss
    - Long-term memory loss
  - Transient somatic side effects
    - Headache, muscle ache, jaw ache
    - Dental fractures, oral trauma, corneal abrasions
  - Arrhythmia—PAC, PVC, nonsustained ventricular tachycardia
    - More common in people with preexisting arrhythmia
    - Typically transient and minor in those without known underlying disease

VAGUS NERVE STIMULATION (VNS)

- **Description:**
  - Initially approved for intractable epilepsy
  - Currently FDA approved for the treatment refractory depression
  - Not commonly used; limited empirical evidence of effectiveness
  - Implanted pulse generator produces electrical stimulation of the left vagus nerve
    - 80% afferent fibers affected
    - Vagus nerve has connections with dorsal raphe, locus coeruleus, thalamus

- **Indications and Target Populations**
  - Depression
    - Can be used as adjunctive treatment for chronic or recurrent symptoms for patients older than age 18 years
    - Indicated if refractory to at least four adequate trials of antidepressant therapy (medication or ECT)
- **Complications:**
  - Surgical complications related to implantation of device:
    - Vagus nerve compression
    - Incision pain or infection
  - Throat pain
  - Shortness of breath (increased risk in people with chronic obstructive pulmonary disease)
  - Vocal cord paralysis: voice alteration or hoarseness
  - Dysphagia
- **Contraindication:** prior left vagotomy

Transcranial Magnetic Stimulation

- **Description**
  - Noninvasive stimulation of the prefrontal cortex through induced magnetic field
  - Can be performed as an outpatient procedure
  - Treatment given approximately 5 days a week for 4 to 6 weeks
- **Indications**
  - Not currently FDA approved for the treatment of any psychiatric disorder
  - Approved for major depressive disorder in Canada and Israel
  - Small but significant effect in RCT for depression and auditory hallucinations
- **Contraindications**
  - Intracranial metal implants
  - History of stroke
  - Pregnancy
  - Poorly controlled migraines
- **Complications**
  - Seizure
  - Scalp pain from stimulation of muscles and nerves
  - Headache
  - Lightheadedness

TABLE 5-34 Pre–Electroconvulsive Therapy Checklist

Medical history: prior complications from ECT or anesthesia **Chest radiography** **ECG** **Imaging** • Spinal films if a spinal disorder is suspected • CT or MRI if a space-occupying lesion is suspected **Laboratory** • Chemistries • CBC with differential • UA with reflex culture and sensitivity	**Assess medications for discontinuation during treatment** • Medications with independent risk of adverse cognitive effects (e.g., lithium, anticholinergics—increased risk of encephalopathy) • Theophylline (risk of post-ECT status epilepticus) • Anticonvulsants and benzodiazepines increase the seizure threshold • Medications that are arrhythmogenic (TCAs, MAOIs) **NPO after midnight before ECT**

CBC, complete blood count; CT, computed tomography; ECT, electroconvulsive therapy; MAOI, monoamine oxidase inhibitor; MRI, magnetic resonance imaging; NPO, nothing by mouth; TCA, tricyclic antidepressant; UA, urinalysis.

Psychotherapy

"Don't just do something, sit there."—Anne Alonso

Basic Principles of Treatment

All modalities of psychotherapy rely on two interrelated goals as a foundation of successful therapy:

- **Establishing a frame:**
  - A frame is a psychic structure through which the therapist and patient interact
  - Components include the physical space in which the appointments take place and the interpersonal boundaries between the patient and therapist (i.e., not maintaining a social relationship outside of therapy). A well-established frame allows for minimal distractions from the therapeutic work
- **Establishing a therapeutic alliance:**
  - A therapeutic alliance is the means through which a therapist hopes to engage with and effect change in a patient
  - Building a therapeutic alliance includes establishing a rapport (connecting to patients without colluding with defenses) in addition to showing empathy
  - Techniques used to develop a therapeutic alliance:
    - Be nonjudgmental about the patient's actions (also referred to as a "neutral posture")
    - Ask open-ended questions (e.g., "Tell me more "or "What might that be about?)
    - Avoid why or yes-or-no questions
    - Use a nonjudgmental stance (requirement for an adequate body of knowledge, to tolerate ambiguity)
    - Listen actively, tolerate silences, attend to body language, observe what you see

Psychotherapy Modalities

Several methodologies are commonly practiced that differ both in their interpretation of symptoms as well as treatment methods:

- Supportive psychotherapy
- Cognitive behavioral therapy (CBT)
- Dialectical behavior therapy
- Behavioral therapy
- Psychodynamic psychotherapy

Supportive Psychotherapy

- **Description:**
  - Version of psychodynamic therapy that follows a dynamic formulation but allows for a more active stance on the part of the therapist in supporting the patient
  - Therapist offers leadership and support and encourages self-care and the pursuit of pleasurable activities
  - Allows the patient to verbalize strong emotions with goal of relieving tension and anxiety
- **Characteristics:**
  - Time frame: can range from a few months (short-term bereavement) to many years (certain personality disorders)
  - Frequency: typically once weekly but can be more frequent
  - Loosely structured, not manualized

Cognitive Behavioral Therapy

- Developed primarily by Aaron Beck and colleagues
- **Description:** tries to change thoughts (cognitions) and behaviors in order to change emotions
- **Target population and disorders:** most often used for depressive disorders but also used for panic disorder, obsessive–compulsive disorder, paranoid personality disorder, and somatoform disorders
- **Characteristics:**
  - Short-term, structured therapy
  - Involves active collaboration between the patient and therapist
  - More didactic than psychodynamic therapy; the therapist explains the link between the patient's symptoms or disorder and thinking, affect, and behavior and provides a full rationale for treatment
  - Requires homework by the patient
- **Key techniques and terms:**
  - **Cognitive triad or triangle:**
    - Representation of the interrelationship between thoughts, feelings, and behaviors
    - Important component of CBT is to recognize each component of the triangle individually and how it affects the other two components
  - **Automatic negative thoughts (cognitive distortions):**
    - Overgeneralizing: believing that if something is true once, it applies to any similar cases

- Selective abstraction: overemphasizing failures and ignoring achievements
- Excessive responsibility: assuming personal causality for all bad things
- Self-referencing: assuming one's bad traits or performance are at the center of everyone's attention
- Catastrophizing: always thinking the worst is going to happen
- Dichotomous thinking ("black-and-white thinking"): thinking everything should be judged at an extreme, either all good or all bad
- **Reality testing:**
  - The patient is asked to recall automatic negative thoughts that came up in a particular situation
  - The patient tests the validity of these thoughts with the goal of demonstrating that their content is inaccurate or exaggerated
  - Alternative, more realistic explanations are generated
- **Core beliefs:** assumptions or rules about the self that often underlie the patient's cognitive distortions
- **Behavioral scheduling:** technique of targeting maladaptive behaviors by having the patient plan out a week's worth of activities by the hour, record whether these activities were done as planned, and the review record with therapist

Dialectical Behavior Therapy (DBT)

- Developed by Marsha Linehan
- **Description:** Adjunctive technique to other psychotherapy techniques; uses supportive, cognitive and behavioral techniques with the goal of improving interpersonal skills and decreasing self-destructive behavior; based on the theory that borderline patients cannot identify emotional experiences or tolerate frustration or rejection
- **Target population and disorders:** patients with borderline personality disorder or parasuicidal behaviors
- **Characteristics:**
  - Time frame: can last up to many years
  - Uses both group and individual therapy
  - Involves homework assignments and coaching, both in person and over the phone
  - Five functions of treatment:
    - Enhance the patient's repertoire of socially adaptive behaviors
    - Improve the patient's motivation to change by reducing reinforcement of maladaptive behaviors
    - Ensure that newly acquired effective behaviors are used in a natural environment
    - Structure the environment so that effective, not dysfunctional, behaviors are reinforced
    - Support the therapist's motivation and capabilities (e.g., through weekly team meeting aimed at enhancing the therapist's skills or preventing burnout)

- **Skills taught in DBT:**
  - Mindfulness: adapted from Buddhist teachings and is related to meditation; focuses on self-awareness of thoughts, actions, or motivation
  - Interpersonal effectiveness: focuses on interpersonal interactions, including actions such as asking for what one needs, saying no, and coping with interpersonal conflict
  - Distress tolerance: ability to accept, in a non-evaluative and nonjudgmental fashion, both oneself and the current situation
  - Emotional regulation: focuses on the control of emotional states and responses to stress

Behavioral Therapy

- Based on the research of B.F. Skinner and others
- **Description:** focuses on verifiable behaviors and their effects on the environment; arose from behaviorism, which believed that only publicly observable behaviors could be studied scientifically (as opposed to mental content such as thoughts and feeling states)
- **Target population and disorders:** individuals with phobias, anxiety disorders, and depression
- **Characteristics:** sessions involve exposing subject over time to uncomfortable stimuli related to the source of their symptoms; treatment is time limited
- **Key techniques:**
  - Systematic desensitization: Uses counterconditioning to reduce the anxiety response to feared things or events by pairing external threatening stimuli with an internal relaxed state; has the patient enter a state of relaxation and then imagine increasingly anxiety-provoking scenes while maintaining the relaxed state; relaxation training methods include progressive relaxation of major muscle groups or mental imagery (picturing oneself in a place associated with calmness and relaxation)
  - Therapeutic graded exposure: similar to systematic desensitization but does not involve relaxation training and uses real-life stimuli instead of imagined scenes
  - Flooding (or imaginal flooding): instead of a hierarchy of increasingly anxiety-provoking stimuli, the patient is exposed in vivo to the feared object and is discouraged from escaping or withdrawing prematurely; the underlying concept is that if the patient has access to escape, the conditioned avoidance behavior would be reinforced; the patient initially experiences intense fear, which subsides, and the patient eventually achieves a feeling of calmness and mastery over the feared stimulus

Psychodynamic Psychotherapy

- **Key features:**
  - Focuses on developmental processes
  - Focuses on transference and counter-transference between patient and therapist
  - Relies on a dynamic unconscious
  - Treatment comes from depth understanding

- **Description**
  - Involves interpretation of unconscious conflict with goal of generating insight
  - May increase anxiety at first as awareness of conflict grows but ultimately enhances patient's self-knowledge and sense of personal agency
  - Depends on a nonjudgmental stance by the therapist to minimize the patient's sense of shame as previously unacknowledged emotions, attitudes, and aspects of the self become known

KEY TECHNIQUES AND TERMS

- **Transference:** Unconscious aspects of emotional relationships with early caregivers are reexperienced with or transferred onto the therapist in the present. The therapist should interpret transference as it emerges, allowing the patient to understand how relational attitudes arising from the past are often painful or traumatic experiences are repeated and how they create difficulties in present relationships
- **Countertransference:** Unconscious feelings experienced by the therapist in working with the patient. Although this is a feature in all dynamic work, it is particularly emphasized in object relations theory, which focuses on how early relationships with important other people are internalized and make up the set of relational attitudes automatically used by a person in subsequent encounters. The therapist's changing feelings are thought to represent reactions to the different relationships that the patient is reenacting with the therapist. Countertransference and transference frequently overlap and interact, creating a dynamic aspect of the mutually constructed treatment relationship
- **Resistance:** An unconscious process used by patients to fend off anxiety and maintain the status quo. Defenses are an attempt to ward off painful affect related to the patient's central conflict. There are many different types of defenses, ranging from more adaptive ones (humor, sublimation) to less adaptive ones (projection, substance use, externalization). Any psychological function can be used as a defense against psychological distress
- **Free association:**
  - Freud's "fundamental rule" of how to conduct psychoanalysis
  - The patient agrees to tell the therapist everything that comes to mind without selection or filtering
  - Encourages the unconscious material to emerge so that the deep conflicts leading to symptom formation can be explored
- **Key techniques:**
  - **Clarification:** technique that asks questions aimed at explaining ambiguities or filling in the gaps in the conscious material of the therapy narrative
  - **Suggestion:** a technique often used in hypnosis whereby the therapist induces an idea without argument or coercion (a key aspect of hypnosis)
  - **Interpretation:** a strategic statement by the therapist that draws a link between the patient's statement and an unconscious process *(continued)*

TABLE 5-35 Schools of Psychoanalytic Teaching

Classic Freudian or Ego Psychology Sigmund Freud, Karl Abraham, Anna Freud, Heinz Hartmann, Edith Jacobson	
Description	Freud's original theory; aims to make unconscious conflicts conscious, thus enhancing the ability to work and love; importance of ego defenses emphasized by later proponents
Concepts	• The unconscious • Dynamic interplay between the id, ego, and superego • Oedipal conflict • Ego defense mechanisms • Eros and thanatos
Technique	• Free association, dream interpretation • Therapist mostly just listens with evenly suspended attention; sometimes offers interpretations • Countertransference considered a "technical error" that needed to be remedied by the psychoanalyst
Object Relations Melanie Klein, Wilfred Bion, Michael Balint, W.R.D. Fairbairn, Donald H. Winnicott, Otto Kernberg	
Description	Early relational attitudes toward others are internalized as "self-objects," informing the set of available rxns to others throughout life; approach aims to integrate split-off, primitively affectively charged self representations into more integrated, flexible, governable experiences of the self
Concepts	• Good breast and bad breast • Self-object dyad • "Good enough" mother and therapist • Holding environment • Transitional object
Technique	• Interpretation makes the patient aware of ambivalent, contradictory feelings (different parts of the self) experienced across time; awareness leads to integration of split-off self-objects • Countertransference in this theory is caused by the patient's projected intrapsychic objects, so it is considered important data
Self-psychology Heinz Kohut	
Description	Parents' failure to empathize with their child leads to "defects" in the child's self, experienced as psychopathology
Concepts	• Empathy • Self-object • Optimal frustration • Mirroring • Twinship • Tripolar self
Technique	• Therapist uses empathy to make the patient feel seen and understood, which leads to a cure

(continued)

- **Dream interpretation:**
  - Thought to be a particularly potent method for bringing repressed material into awareness
  - Conceptualized by Freud as an unconscious wish repressed since childhood transformed into the content and imagery of dreams by condensation and displacement
  - Recent findings from neuroscience seem to confirm the adaptive function of dreams for psychological well-being
- **Defense mechanism:** the mind is adept at keeping the unconscious conflictual material out of awareness using a variety of psychological defenses; these can be psychotic, immature, neurotic, or normal, in order from least to most socially adaptive

TABLE 5-36 A Brief Sample of the Psychological Defense Mechanisms

Defense	Level	Description
Delusional projection	I, psychotic	Fixed, false beliefs about external reality, usually of a persecutory nature
Example: a patient raised in a setting of chronic physical and sexual abuse is filled with unacknowledged murderous rage; this rage is delusionally projected onto the "CIA," which she believes is pursuing her in order to kill her		
Denial	I, psychotic	Refusal to accept what is clearly going on in reality because it is too threatening
Example: a soldier's arm is blown off in combat, but in a state of terror, he refuses to acknowledge that the limb is missing		
Projection	II, immature	Attributing one's own unacknowledged unacceptable or unwanted thoughts and emotions to another
Example: a patient had an always hypercritical, even sadistic mother; he makes stinging remarks to his wife, provoking her to react angrily and vindictively; he calls her the angry one (the projection), not seeing that his own unacknowledged angry acts elicit her responses		
Repression	III, neurotic	Painful or dangerous thoughts are automatically prevented from entering the consciousness, although a painful emotion is still felt
Example: a patient is terrified of heights; she has repressed a hatred of and wish to kill her alcoholic mother so she could have her idealized father all to herself; being high up elicits anxiety, the conflictual emotional trace of the desired but guilt-ridden triumph		
Sublimation	IV, normal	Transformation of negative emotions or instincts into positive actions, behavior, or emotion
Example: a patient who recovered from a childhood cancer sublimates his fear of sickness into the drive necessary to complete a rigorous medical training and become an oncologist		

TABLE 5-37 Example of Interpretation

Passive–aggressive acts toward the therapist such as showing up late for the appointment or not paying the bill on time may reflect repressed murderous rage toward an abusive parent. After the therapist is convinced of a link, the transference act should be quickly interpreted so that it does not intensify, potentially destroying the treatment. Not brought into awareness by interpretation, the murderous rage might soon express itself by the patient's abruptly leaving treatment, in effect "killing" the therapy.

REFERENCES

The collected papers of Paul Libbey Russell, MDH. *Smith College Studies in Social Work* 2006, 76(1/2).

Freud S. Recommendations for physicians on the psychoanalytic method of treatment. *Collected Papers,* vol 2. New York: Basic Books; 1912:323–333.

Gabbard G, ed. *Core Competencies in Psychotherapy Series* (5 volumes). Washington, DC: American Psychiatric Publishing; 2004.

Luborsky L. *Principles of Psychoanalytic Psychotherapy: A Manual for Supportive-Expressive Treatment.* New York: Basic Books; 1984.

MacKinnon RA, Michels R, Buckley PJ. *The Psychiatric Interview in Clinical Practice.* Philadelphia: WB Saunders; 1971.

Steven S. *Essential Psychopharmacology: The Prescriber's Guide.* New York: Cambridge University Press; 2004.

Wachtel P. *Relational Theory and the Practice of Psychotherapy.* New York: The Guilford Press; 2008.

Wachtel P. *Therapeutic Communication: Knowing What To Say When.* New York: The Guilford Press; 1993.

Chapter 6

CLINICAL REFERENCES

General Neurology

NEUROANATOMY

- **Cerebral cortex:** convoluted sheet of neural tissue at the rostral pole of the neuraxis; functionally includes the hippocampus

TABLE 6-1 Regions of the Cerebral Cortex

	Function	Input	Blood Supply
Occipital lobe	Visual	LGN thalamus	PCA
Temporal lobe	Visual form perception (lateral, inferior) Audition and language (superior) Memory (medial)	MGN thalamus, occipital and frontal cortices	MCA
Parietal lobe	Visual motion, space perception, somatosensation, polysensory processing, visuospatial attention, movement planning, language (dominant hemisphere)	VP and pulvinar thalamus, occipital and frontal cortices	MCA
Frontal lobe	Movement planning and execution, memory, executive function, awareness, insight, judgment Speech (lateral, dominant hemisphere)	VL and medial dorsal thalamus	MCA, ACA
Limbic system*	Memory, emotion, motivation, visceral processing (autonomic, gustatory, endocrine)	Papez circuit†	ACA, MCA

*The limbic system consists of the hippocampus, amygdala, septum, cingulate, orbital, insula, hypothalamus, and mamillary bodies.

†Papez circuit: cingulate → parahippocampal gyrus → hippocampus → fornix → mammillary bodies → anterior thalamus → cingulate.

ACA, anterior cerebral artery; MCA, middle cerebral artery; LGN, lateral geniculate nucleus; MGN, medial geniculate nucleus; PCA, posterior cerebral artery; VL, ventral lateral; VP, ventral posterior.

- **Cerebellum:**
  - Movement coordination, sensory–motor integration, balance, modulation of affect and cognition
  - Divided into lateral hemispheres, medial vermis, flocculonodular lobe, and deep cerebellar nuclei (dentate, interpositus, fastigial, and vestibular)
  - Blood supply is from the superior cerebellar artery (SCA), anterior inferior cerebellar artery (AICA), posterior inferior cerebellar artery (PICA)
- **Basal ganglia:** caudate, putamen, globus pallidus, nucleus accumbens, subthalamic nucleus and substantia nigra
  - Motor control, cognition, emotion, learning
  - Direct pathway (stimulatory): → globus pallidus interna (GPi) and substantia nigra pars reticulata (SNr) → thalamus → cortex, D1-receptor mediated
  - Indirect pathway (inhibitory): → globus pallidus externa (GPe) → STN → GPi and SNr → thalamus → cortex, D2-receptor mediated
  - Blood supply is mainly from the medial cerebral artery (MCA) (lenticulostriate)
- **Brainstem:** cranial nerve nuclei, midbrain, pons, medulla
  - Integrative functions (cardiovascular, respiratory, pain sensitivity, alertness, sleep–wake cycles)
  - Blood supply is from the direct branches off the basilar, vertebral arteries

TABLE 6-2 Diffuse Modulatory Neurotransmitter Systems

Neurotransmitter	Synthesis Location	Receptors or CNS Pathways	Functions (Example of Pathology)
Cholinergic (ACh)	Basal nucleus of Meynert, medial septal nucleus	M1; brainstem, neocortex, and hippocampus	Learning, short-term memory, arousal, reward (delirium)
Dopaminergic (DA)	Substantia nigra, ventral tegmental area	Mesocortical (dorsolateral prefrontal cortex)	Cognition, motivation (schizophrenia)
		Mesolimbic (nucleus accumbens)	Reward (addiction)
		Nigrostriatal (basal ganglia)	Motor (Parkinson's disease)
		Tuberoinfundibular (hypothalamus)	Prolactin secretion, endocrine function
Noradrenergic (NE)	Locus ceruleus, lateral tegmental area	Receptors diffusely throughout CNS	Arousal, reward, attention (depression, ADHD)
Serotonergic (5HT)	Raphe nuclei	Receptors diffusely throughout CNS	Mood, satiety, temperature, sleep, pain sensitivity (depression, chronic pain symptoms)

ADHD, attention-deficit hyperactivity disorder; CNS, central nervous system.

NEUROLOGIC EXAMINATION FINDINGS

See page 7 for approach to the examination.

Abnormal Speech

- **Dysarthria:** pure motor dysfunction of larynx or tongue
- **Aphasia:** dysfunction in repetition, comprehension, or fluency

TABLE 6-3 Types of Abnormal Speech

Type of Aphasia	Repetition	Comprehension	Fluency
Broca's	Impaired	Intact	Nonfluent
Wernicke's	Impaired	Impaired	Fluent
Conduction	Impaired	Intact	Fluent
Global	Impaired	Impaired	Nonfluent
Transcortical, sensory	Intact	Impaired	Fluent
Transcortical, motor	Intact	Intact	Nonfluent

Abnormal Movements

- **Athetosis:** slow, writhing continuous movements; often brought out by moving other body parts
- **Asterixis:** transient lapses of limb postural control, most often caused by hepatic or renal failure
- **Chorea:** involuntary, irregular, purposeless, nonrhythmic, abrupt movements that flow from one body part to another; increased by stress; caused by caudate nucleus damage from streptococcal infection (Sydenham's chorea), Huntington's disease, drugs, or systemic lupus erythematosus
- **Dyskinesia:** abnormal involuntary movement (vs. **tardive dyskinesia,** which are involuntary, continuous movements clustered around the mouth and face, usually caused by long-term antipsychotic or levodopa use)
- **Dystonia:** twisting movements; sustained at peak of the movement; repetitive and often progressing to prolonged abnormal postures; caused by co-contraction of agonist or antagonist muscles; focal dystonias include blepharospasm (eyelids), spasmodic torticollis (neck), oculogyric crisis (eyes), buccolingual crisis (mouth or tongue)
- **Hemiballismus:** large-amplitude choreiform movements; usually from a lesion of the contralateral subthalamic nucleus
- **Myoclonus:** brief, irregular movement of the muscles; cannot be controlled by effort or will (unlike tics); may be repetitive; generalized myoclonus occurs in familial disorder, subacute sclerosing panencephalitis, Creutzfeldt-Jakob disease, toxic metabolic encephalopathy
- **Tics:** repetitive, stereotyped movements (motor or vocal) under some degree of voluntary control
  - **Tourette's syndrome:** chronic tic disorder beginning before age 18 years; tics occur multiple times per day for more than1 year; treatment includes

clonidine, guanfacine, antipsychotics (especially Pimozide), selective serotonin reuptake inhibitors (especially if the patient has comorbid depression or obsessive–compulsive symptoms); habit reversal therapy, and surgery (deep brain stimulation for severe refractory disease); psychostimulants may exacerbate tics

- **Tremor:**
  - **Resting:** idiopathic; seen in Parkinson's disease (3–6 Hz); decreases with movement; treatment: anticholinergics, dopamine agonists, amantadine, levodopa
  - **Action:** physiologic; postural (8–12 Hz); enhanced with nebulizers, anxiety, caffeine, endocrine disorders
  - **Essential:** recurrent constant tremor of the arms or head (4–8 Hz) may be kinetic or postural, autosomal dominant; improves with alcohol; treatment: propranolol, primidone, topiramate stereotactic surgery or stimulation
  - **Orthostatic:** appears after minutes of standing; treatment; clonazepam
  - **Drug-induced:** antipsychotics, antidepressants, levodopa, beta agonists, lithium, caffeine, amphetamines, steroids

---

Neurologic Illnesses

Ischemic Stroke

RISK FACTORS

- **Modifiable:** hypertension (HTN), cardiac disease, hyperlipidemia, tobacco, diabetes mellitus, obstructive sleep apnea, physical inactivity, carotid artery stenosis, use of oral contraceptives (especially in smokers), drug use (cocaine, heroin, alcohol), treatable prothrombotic states (e.g., cancers, infections)
- **Nonmodifiable:** Age (>55 years), race (African American, Hispanic > Caucasian), family history, prior stroke or transient ischemic attack, heritable coagulopathies

CAUSES

- Cardioembolic: 20% (roughly 50% associated with atrial fibrillation)
- Small vessel disease: 25%
- Large vessel disease: 20%
- Cryptogenic: 30%
- Other: 5% (hypercoagulable states, dissections, arteritis, migraine or vasospasm, drug abuse)

Large Vessel Acute Stroke Syndromes

- **Middle cerebral artery (MCA):** Contralateral motor and sensory loss with aphasia (dominant) or neglect (nondominant)
- **Anterior cerebral artery (ACA):** unilateral → contralateral lower extremity weakness; bilateral → bilateral lower extremity weakness, bladder symptoms, abulia
- **Posterior cerebral artery (PCA):** homonymous hemianopsia, memory loss, language dysfunction, hemisensory loss or hemiplegia, visual agnosia
- **Vertebral artery (VA):** altered gait, dizziness, lateral medullary symptoms (Horner's syndrome, ipsilateral ataxia, contralateral hypoalgesia, ipsilateral cranial nerve V palsy, nystagmus)

- **Unilateral ICA:** amaurosis fugax, hemiparesis, hemianopsia, aphasia (dominant side), hemineglect (nondominant side), Horner's syndrome
- **Anterior ACA or MCA:** crural hemiparesis with mutism, transcortical motor aphasia (dominant side) or mood change (nondominant side)
- **Posterior MCA and PCA:** hemianopia with transcortical sensory aphasia (dominant side) or neglect (nondominant side)
  - Subcortical (cortical and deep MCA branches): hemiparesis and stepwise progression
- **Watershed infarcts:** ischemic infarction in a territory located at the periphery of two bordering arterial distributions

Transient Ischemic Attack

- **Symptoms:** clear onset (usually <1 min) and course (usually <20 min; maximum, 24 hr)
- **Differential diagnosis:** migraines, focal seizure, tumors, subdural hematoma (SDH), hypoglycemia, primary ear or eye disease

Hemorrhage

INTERCEREBRAL HEMORRHAGE (HEMORRHAGIC STROKE)

- **Causes:** HTN (most common), aneurysm or arteriovenous malformation (AVM) rupture, trauma, coagulopathy (thrombocytopenia, liver disease, leukemia, aplastic anemia, anticoagulant or thrombolytic treatment), central nervous system (CNS) tumors (primary or metastatic), septic emboli, vasculitis, amyloid angiopathy, use of vasopressor drugs, exertion, herpes encephalitis

SUBARACHNOID HEMORRHAGE

- **Causes:** trauma (most common), aneurysm, AVM, angiopathies (Marfan syndrome, polycystic kidney disease, Ehlers-Danlos), coagulopathies, venous thrombosis, allergic reaction, meningitis, herpes encephalitis, drugs (cocaine, amphetamines), brain tumors, eclampsia, vasculitis
- **Symptoms:** sudden-onset, severe headache ("worst headache of my life"); brief loss of consciousness (LOC); lethargy; somnolence; meningeal signs; nausea and vomiting; focal neurologic symptoms (may be absent); HTN; retinal hemorrhages

Seizures

- **Generalized seizures:** result in abnormal activity throughout the cortex; LOC; usually no aura or specific warning; may have a nonspecific prodrome
  - **Generalized tonic-clonic seizures:** LOC; tonic contractions followed by symmetric limb jerks followed by postictal phase; look for Todd's paralysis (focal neurologic deficit that resolves over 36 hours)
  - **Absence seizures:** genetically transmitted; start in childhood and rare after puberty; spells with brief LOC (5–10 sec) with no loss of tone; also have subtle motor signs and automatisms; patients have hundreds of spells daily
  - **Other generalized seizures:**
    - **Tonic seizures:** continued muscle contraction with LOC; may lead to arrest of ventilation; may lead to a fall and drop attack

  - **Clonic seizures:** clonic jerking with LOC
  - **Myoclonic seizures:** sudden, brief, shocklike contractions; localized or generalized
  - **Atonic seizures:** result from loss of postural tone; lead to a fall and drop attack
- **Partial seizures:** localized in one area of the brain; also called focal
  - **Simple partial seizures:** consciousness is unaffected; may then generalize; **Jacksonian march**—spread to contiguous reasons of the motor cortex
  - **Complex partial seizures:** consciousness is altered; most common type in adults; commonly associated with neuropsychiatric phenomena; usually arise from temporal or frontal lobe; automatism may be present
    - **Temporal lobe epilepsy:** aura with olfactory or other hallucinations, hyperreligiosity, macropsia, micropsia, déjà vu, jamais vu, dissociative symptoms, unprovoked panic
    - **Frontal lobe epilepsy:** behavioral alteration; brief or rapidly generalizing automatisms
    - **Parietal lobe epilepsy:** contralateral sensory deficits; often associated with eye movements and motor activity
    - **Occipital epilepsy:** elementary visual hallucinations (flashes, pulsating light) or formed visual hallucinations, vomiting, migraine, eye movement, with or without focal motor seizure
- **Nonepileptic seizures (NES):** abnormal movements as the result of another medical or neurologic problem or as a result of psychological factors
  - Common; seen in 10% of patients with a seizure disorder, 25% of patients with NES also have true seizures
  - Associated with general medical conditions, deception, and unconscious production of symptoms of epileptic seizures

SPECIAL CONSIDERATIONS

- Discontinue drugs that lower seizure threshold, including clozapine, olanzapine, clomipramine, bupropion, and quetiapine

Neuroimaging

Magnetic Resonance Imaging (MRI)

- Measures proton spin relaxation parameters (T1, T2) after excitation by radiofrequency (RF) pulses; better than computed tomography (CT) for evaluation of brain anatomy

TABLE 6-4 Types of Magnetic Resonance Imaging

Image Type	Cerebrospinal Fluid	Fat	Utility
T1	Dark	Bright	Anatomy
T2	Bright	Dark	Pathology
FLAIR	Dark	Gray	Pathology (edema, infarct)

- **Gadolinium:** intravenous (IV) contrast to evaluate for enhancement in MS (active lesions), tumors, vascular abnormalities, inflammation
- **Diffusion weighted:** restricted diffusion appears bright as early as 30 min after stroke
- **T2 or gradient echo:** weighted to show deoxy Hgb, iron deposits; best for evaluating presence of blood with MRI
- **Magnetic resonance angiography (MRA) and venography (MRV):** IV contrast or "time-of-flight" (noncontrast) to evaluate vascular flow

Computed Tomography (CT)

- Measures differential absorption of x-rays
- Better than MRI for acute evaluation of intracranial anatomy, bone, blood, cerebrospinal fluid (CSF) spaces
- Faster, less expensive, and better tolerated than MRI
- Not as good for the brainstem and posterior fossa
- Epidural hematoma: biconvex, limited by sutures, acute
- Subdural hematoma: crescent shaped, crosses sutures, subacute
- Subarachnoid hemorrhage: air-fluid level in ventricles; hyperdensity between sulci and in cisternal spaces

Positron Emission Tomography (PET)

- Measures emission of positrons from radionuclides (typically sugars) injected into the bloodstream and taken up by metabolically active tissue
- Provides a measure of metabolic activity; useful in epilepsy localization and in assessing tumor activity
- Slow, requires invasive tracer, typically low spatial resolution

Single-Proton Emission Computed Tomography (SPECT)

- Similar to PET but measures protons instead of positrons
- Used to visualize metabolic changes that can help to distinguish different types of dementia

Electroencephalography (EEG)

- Electrical activity recorded on multiple standardized locations on the scalp to measure electrical activity generated in cerebral cortex and synchronized and modulated by the thalamus and reticular activating system
- Used to confirm, localize, and classify seizures; a normal EEG does not rule out seizure

General Medicine Reference

BASIC LABORATORY STUDIES AND THEIR UTILITY

Chemistries (Chem 7, Chem 10, BMP or CMP)

ROUTINE LABORATORY STUDIES

Ordered for admission or medical clearance

- Chemistries
- Complete blood count
- Beta-HCG (for all woman of childbearing age)
- Urine toxicology
- Psychotropic drug levels

- **When to order:** medical clearance for psychiatric admission; to rule out a metabolic cause of altered mental status; to obtain baseline values before initiating psychiatric medications
- **Specific considerations:**
  - Na: hyponatremia
    - Syndrome of inappropriate antidiuretic hormone secretion (SIADH): inappropriately concentrated urine (Uosm >100); low blood urea nitrogen (BUN) and uric acid; caused by use of certain drugs (oxcarbazepine, antipsychotics, antidepressants), hypothyroidism, pulmonary pathology, intracranial pathology, small cell lung cancer
    - Psychogenic polydipsia: intake of more than 12 to 20 L/day of water; Uosm less than 100 L/day of water; low uric acid
  - Na: hypernatremia
    - Diabetes insipidus (DI): polyuria and polydipsia; ADH absent (central) or has no effect (nephrogenic); lithium can cause nephrogenic DI
  - Creatinine (Cr): may be increased in patients on lithium (kidney damage may occur with long-term use)
  - Glucose: monitor in patients on atypical antipsychotics because of their increased risk for diabetes
    - Fasting glucose above 126 mg/dL or random glucose above 200 mg/dl should prompt further workup
  - K/Mg: replete to normal values, especially in patients at risk for seizure or arrhythmia (e.g., alcohol withdrawal or antipsychotics with QTc prolongation)

Complete Blood Count with or without Differential (CBC +/− Diff)

- **When to order:** medical clearance for psychiatric admission; to rule out infectious cause for altered mental status; to obtain baseline values before initiating psychiatric medications and every 3 to 6 months thereafter
- **Specific considerations:**
  - Monitoring of absolute neutrophil count (ANC) on clozapine
  - Monitoring platelets while the patient is taking valproic acid

Liver Function Tests (LFTs)

- **When to order:** history of alcohol use; suspicion of overdose (e.g., acetaminophen); toxins, hepatitis, or use of valproic acid; to obtain baseline values before initiating antipsychotics or mood stabilizers and every 3 to 6 months thereafter

- **Specific considerations:**
  - Predominantly increased aminotransferases (aspartate aminotransferase [AST] and alanine aminotransferase [ALT]) indicate hepatocellular injury
    - AST:ALT > 2:1 in alcoholic hepatitis
    - ALT > AST in viral hepatitis

Coagulation Profile (coags)

- **When to order:** for patients on warfarin treatment; long history of alcohol use; acetaminophen overdose; advanced liver disease

Thyroid Function Tests (TFTs)

- **When to order:** initial workup of depression or anxiety; before initiating treatment with and every 6 months while on lithium
- **Symptoms of hypothyroidism:** weight gain, fatigue, myalgias, arthralgias, depression, menorrhagia, constipation, dry skin or nails, delayed deep tendon reflexes, carpal tunnel syndrome
- **Symptoms of hyperthyroidism:** weight loss, restlessness, tachycardia, palpitations, heat intolerance, increased frequency of bowel movements, sweating, moist skin or nails; proptosis and goiter in Graves' disease
- **Thyroid-stimulating hormone (TSH):** most sensitive test to detect primary hypo- and hyperthyroidism; may be inappropriately normal with central causes
- If TSH is abnormal, check free thyroxine (T4) level and refer the patient for further evaluation

Urinalysis (U/A)

- **When to order:** medical clearance for geriatric psychiatry admission; to rule out urinary tract infection (UTI) or urosepsis as the cause of altered mental status; for suspected diabetic ketoacidosis (DKA) or eating disorders; concern for rhabdomyolysis
- **Notes on interpretation:**
  - Increased white blood (WBC) cell count (leukocyte esterase) indicates inflammation (UTI, glomerular nephritis, interstitial nephritis); order urine culture
  - Nitrites suggest *Enterobacteriaceae* UTI; order urine culture
  - Increased red blood cell (RBC) count indicates glomerulonephritis, nephrolithiasis, urinary tract malignancy or trauma; also with microglobinuria in rhabdomyolysis (e.g., cocaine, seizure, neuroleptic malignant syndrome, extreme muscular exertion)
  - Ketones are present in ketoacidosis (e.g., DKA, poor oral intake)

Urine Toxicology (Utox)

See page 34 for more information.

Serum Toxicology (Stox)

- Useful in suspected overdose or when determination of specific substances of use or abuse is indicated (e.g., alprazolam rather than benzodiazepines)

- Often includes ethanol, methanol, acetaminophen, and aspirin
- Contact the individual laboratory to determine which specific assays are available

Lumbar Puncture (LP) and CSF Findings

- **When to order:** altered mental status or seizure with fever, headache, stiff neck, photophobia
- Evaluate for meningitis, encephalitis, neurosyphilis, other CNS infections, subarachnoid hemorrhage, multiple sclerosis; high-volume LP is both diagnostic and therapeutic in normal-pressure hydrocephalous
  - Elderly patients with meningitis may not have a fever
- Obtain CT scan before LP in patients with focal neurologic findings because LP in individuals with mass lesions may precipitate herniation.

TABLE 6-5 Cerebrospinal Findings in Meningitis

	Appearance	Pressure (mm Hg)	WBC/mm³ Predominant Type	Glucose (mg/dL)	Total Protein (mg/dL)
Normal	Clear	9–18	0–5 lymphocytes	50–75	15–40
Bacterial	Cloudy	18–30	100–10,000 polymorphone-ucleated cells	<45	100–1000
	Cloudy	18–30	<500 lymphocytes	<45	100–200
Fungal	Cloudy	18–30	<300 lymphocytes	<45	40–300
	Clear	9–18	<300 polys → lymphocytes	50–100	50–100

WBC, white blood cell.

ELECTROCARDIOGRAPHY (EKG OR ECG)

When to Order

- Medical clearance for geriatric psychiatry admission
- Symptomatic patients: chest pain, palpitations
- Patients at high risk: coronary artery disease, hypertension, diabetes
- Cocaine use (and symptomatic)
- Baseline before initiation of antipsychotics and every 3 to 6 months thereafter

Systemic Interpretation of the ECG

REVIEW

- Entire ECG to obtain and overview and note any obvious abnormalities
- Frontal plane axis
- Rate of ventricles (QRS) and atria (P)

- Rhythm (regular, irregular)
- Relation of P waves to QRS complexes
- Morphology of all complexes (P, QRS, ST-T)
- Intervals (P-R, QT)
- For abnormalities such as Wolff-Parkinson-White (short PR, delta waves)

QTc PROLONGATION

- Baseline and periodic follow-up are recommended for patients receiving tricyclic antidepressants (TCAs), thioridazine, pimozide, chlorpromazine, mesoridazine, ziprasidone, and high-dose IV haloperidol
- QTc: QT interval corrected for heart rate, calculated by:

$$QTc = \frac{QT}{\sqrt{(RR)}}$$

  - QTc prolongation (>440 ms) is an independent risk factor for sudden death from cardiac arrest
  - Arizona CERT (www.qtdrugs.org) maintains an updated listing of drugs associated with QT prolongation

TRICYCLIC ANTIDEPRESSANTS: CARDIOLOGY AND ELECTROCARDIOGRAPHIC EFFECTS

- Prolong ventricular depolarization, lengthening the PR and QRS intervals as well as QTc
- Act like class IA antiarrhythmic drugs such as quinidine and procainamide (so patients with premature ventricular contractions may improve on TCAs)
- Use in arrhythmias beyond first-degree heart block should be coordinated with cardiology and require K and Mg repletion

APPENDIX I: How to Read a Study

Assessing the importance and validity of the outcomes of a study requires a careful reading of the report. When reading a journal article, address each section in the order below and be able to answer these questions at the end of each section.

TITLE AND ABSTRACT

Identifies the focus of the study and allows readers to decide if reading the entire article is worthwhile

- What is the purpose of the study, and is the purpose clearly stated?
- What is the major finding of the work?
- Is the population studied relevant or comparable to your own clinical population?
- Are the results statistically significant? Clinically significant?

INTRODUCTION

Provides background information relevant to the field and states the context of the hypothesis being tested; may be skimmed or skipped if you are very familiar with the field

- How does the current study relate to previous work in the field?
- Is the current study a valuable and novel contribution to the field?

MATERIALS AND METHODS

Provides a detailed description of how each aspect of the study was conducted

- Is the study design appropriate to the question being addressed? Is it capable of providing useful results?
- Are the time-course of the study and its follow-up appropriate?
- Are the criteria for inclusion and exclusion made clear? Can the results be generalized beyond the studied population?
- Were the subjects randomized among groups? Is the method for randomization adequately described?
- Are the statistical methods adequately described and appropriate for the study?
- Is the power of the study addressed?

RESULTS

Offers detailed description of the study findings and their initial interpretation

- Do the findings address the research questions stated in the introduction?
- Are the groups being compared adequately similar in demographics?
- Do the authors provide actual data for the reader to evaluate or only their own analysis of the data?
- What statistical measures were used to evaluate the data, and are those measures appropriate?
- Do you as the reader have an adequate understanding of the way the findings are formulated (e.g., number needed to treat (NNT), number needed to harm (NNH)) to objectively assess their clinical significance?

DISCUSSION

Provides the author's interpretation of the findings of the work and the relevance of those findings to the larger field

- Are the conclusions justified? Are they relevant to your practice?
- How do the findings relate to established practice and previous studies?
- Was the study worthwhile? Does it make a valuable contribution to the field?
- Do the authors address the shortcomings of the work?
  - ***P* value:** the probability of observing an outcome as extreme as the one that was obtained if the null hypothesis is true, or the probability that the observed outcome could have occurred by chance alone. The *P* value accepted as statistically significant is set at ≤ 0.05 by convention

TABLE 6-6 Study Designs in Medical Research

Study Design	Description	Useful for Identifying	Strengths	Weaknesses
Observational Studies				
Case series	An uncontrolled description of an interesting finding observed in a small number of patients	Hypotheses for further study	Can be performed with little preexisting knowledge of the disorder Simple to execute	Usually not hypothesis driven Usually not controlled
Case-control or retrospective studies	Cases with a particular outcome are contrasted with control cases lacking that outcome in an attempt to identify risk factors	Risk factors, causes, and incidence of disease	Useful in study of rare conditions and protracted risk factors	Usually not hypothesis driven Highly prone to bias
Cross-sectional or prevalence studies	The prevalence of an outcome as well as other characteristics of a defined population are assessed at a single point in time	Disease processes, diagnosis, and staging strategies	Relatively inexpensive and simple to perform	Cannot establish causal relations
Cohort studies	A prospective or retrospective study of a chosen population to determine the association between an identified exposure and a particular outcome	Risk factors, prognosis, natural history, and incidence of disease	Observes subjects over long time scale Low recall bias	Expensive Time intensive High attrition rates

(continued)

TABLE 6-6 Study Designs in Medical Research (*continued*)

Study Design	Description	Useful for Identifying	Strengths	Weaknesses
Experimental Studies				
Randomized, controlled trial	A prospective study of subjects randomly assigned to receive one of multiple interventions to determine the relationship between the intervention and the outcome	Treatment efficacy, treatment side effect profile	Provides the strongest level of evidence for causation Least susceptible to bias	May not be possible or ethical in all cases Expensive
Nonrandomized trial	As above without randomization of subjects	Treatment efficacy, treatment side effect profile	Randomization may not always be possible	Prone to bias
Trial with external controls	Subjects receive an intervention, and the outcome is compared with data from a previous study	Treatment efficacy, treatment side effect profile	Creating a proper control group may be difficult for ethical or practical reasons Reduced study expense	Comparison with controls is questionable Prone to bias
Uncontrolled study	A study in which all subjects receive the same intervention and are then followed to observe their outcomes	Treatment side effect profile	May be the most ethically sound design option in some situations	Technically not an experimental study Prone to type I error
Meta-Analyses				
Meta-analysis	Study that analyzes the results of several previous studies that address related hypotheses	Conclusive evidence in areas where previous studies were conflicting or of low power	Greater power than individual studies Protects against overinterpreting differences across studies	Subject to the bias present in the studies being analyzed

APPENDIX II: Abnormal Involuntary Movement Scale (AIMS)

INDICATIONS

- Developed as screening tool for tardive dyskinesia (TD) and for periodic follow-up of those diagnosed with TD
- Should be performed before initiation of neuroleptic treatment and every 6 months thereafter or more frequently if previously undetected movements are noted or with significant change in medication dose

BEFORE BEGINNING

- Observe the patient unobtrusively at rest
- Ask the patient if there is anything in his or her mouth (e.g., gum) and, if so, ask him or her to remove it
- Ask the patient about the *current* condition of his or her teeth. Ask the patient if he or she wears dentures. Ask the patient if his or her teeth or dentures bother the patient *now*
- Ask the patient whether he or she notices any movement in the mouth, face, hands, or feet. If yes, ask the patient to describe and indicate to what extent this movement *currently* bothers the patient or interferes with his or her activities

SCORING

- After observing the patient, rate movements on a scale of 0 (none), 1 (minimal), 2 (mild), 3 (moderate), and 4 (severe)
- When rating movement severity, consider its quality, frequency, and amplitude
- Severity can be assessed in two complementary ways: by global severity score (item 8) and total severity score (sum of items 1–7)

INSTRUCTIONS

1. Have the patient sit in chair with the hands on the knees, legs slightly apart, and feet flat on the floor. Look at the entire body for movements while the patient is in this position
2. Ask the patient to sit with the hands hanging unsupported. If the patient is male, he should place his hands between his legs; if the patient is female and wearing a dress, she should place her hands hanging over her knees. Observe the patient's hands and other body areas
3. Ask the patient to open his or her mouth. Observe the tongue at rest within the mouth. Do this twice
4. Ask the patient to protrude his or her tongue. Observe abnormalities of tongue movement. Do this twice
5. Ask the patient to tap his or her thumb with each finger as rapidly as possible for 10 to 15 seconds, separately with the right hand and then with the left hand. Observe the patient's facial and leg movements
6. Flex and extend the patient's left and right arms

(*continued*)

TABLE 6-7 Modified Abnormal Involuntary Movement Scale

Instructions	Complete examination procedure before making ratings For movement ratings, rate highest severity observed	0 = None 1 = Minimal 2 = Mild 3 = Moderate 4 = Severe
Facial and oral movements	1. Muscles of facial expression: movements of forehead, eyebrows, periorbital area; include frowning, blinking, grimacing	0 1 2 3 4
	2. Lips and perioral area: puckering, pouting, smacking	0 1 2 3 4
	3. Jaw: biting, clenching, chewing, mouth opening, lateral movement	0 1 2 3 4
	4. Tongue: rate only increase in movement both in and out of mouth, not the inability to sustain movement	0 1 2 3 4
Extremity movements	5. Upper (arms, wrists, hands, fingers): choreic (rapid, objectively purposeless, irregular, spontaneous) and athetoid (slow, irregular, complex, serpentine); don not include tremor (repetitive, regular, rhythmic)	0 1 2 3 4
	6. Lower (legs, knees, ankles): lateral knee movement, foot tapping, heel dropping, foot squirming, inversion or eversion of the foot	0 1 2 3 4
Trunk movements	7. Neck, shoulders, hips, rocking, twisting, squirming, pelvic gyrations, including diaphragmatic movements	0 1 2 3 4
Global judgments	8. Severity of abnormal movements	0 1 2 3 4
	9. Incapacitation because of abnormal movements	0 1 2 3 4
	10. Patient's awareness of abnormal movements	0 1 2 3 4
Dental status	11. Current problems with teeth or dentures?	No = 0 Yes = 1
	12. Does the patient usually wear dentures?	No = 0 Yes = 1

Adapted from Munetz MR, Benjamin S: How to examine patients using the abnormal involuntary movements scale. *Hosp Commun Psychiatry* 1988;39(11):1172–1177.

(continued)

7. Ask the patient to stand up. Observe in the patient profile. Observe all body areas again, including the hips.
8. Ask the patient to extend both arms outstretched in front with the palms down. Observe the patient's trunk, legs, and mouth.
9. Have the patient walk a few paces, turn, and walk back to the chair. Observe the patient's hands and gait. Do this twice.

APPENDIX III

TABLE 6-8 Selected Cytochrome P450 Isoenzyme Substrates, Inhibitors, and Inducers

Enzyme	Substrates	Inhibitors	Inducers
1A2	Acetaminophen, caffeine, clozapine, cyclobenzamine, estradiol, fluvoxamine, haloperidol, mirtazapine, ondansetron, olanzapine, phenacetin, procarcinogens, propranolol ramelteon, roprinole, tacrine, TCAs, theophylline, verapamil, warfarin, zolmitriptan	Amiodarone, cimetidine, fluoroquinolones, fluvoxamine, grapefruit juice, methoxsalen, ticlopidine	Charbroiled meats, tobacco (cigarette smoking), cruciferous vegetables, modafinil, omeprazole
2C	Barbiturates, diazepam, fluvastatin, glipizide, glyburide, irbesartan losartan, mephenytoin, NSAIDs, nelfinavir, phenytoin, primidone, propranolol, proguanil, PPIs, rosiglitazone, tamoxifen, tertiary TCAs, THC, r-warfarin, s-warfarin	Fluoxetine, fluvoxamine, ketoconazole, modafinil, omeprazole, oxcarbazepine, sertraline	Carbamazepine, norethindrone, prednisone, rifampin, secobarbital
2D6	Aripiprazole, atomoxetine, beta-blockers (lipophilic), codeine, debrisoquine, dextromethorphan, diltiazem, donepezil, duloxetine, encainide, flecainide, haloperidol, hydroxycodone, lidocaine, metoclopramide, mexiletine, mCPP, nifedipine, ondansetron, phenothiazines (e.g., thioridazine, perphenazine) promethazine, propafenone, risperidone, SSRIs, tamoxifen, TCAs, tramadol, trazodone, venlafaxine	Amiodarone, anti-malarials, bupropion, cimetidine, citalopram, duloxetine, escitalopram, fluoxetine, methadone, metoclopramide, moclobemide, paroxetine, phenothiazines, protease inhibitors, quinidine, sertraline, terbinafine, TCAs, yohimbine	Dexamethasone, rifampin

(continued)

TABLE 6-8 Selected Cytochrome P450 Isoenzyme Substrates, Inhibitors, and Inducers (*continued*)

Enzyme	Substrates	Inhibitors	Inducers
3A3/4	Alfentanil, alprazolam, amiodarone, amprenavir, aripiprazole, bromocriptine, buspirone, Cafergot, CCBs, caffeine, carbamazepine, cisapride, clozapine, cyclosporine, dapsone, diazepam, disopyramide, efavirenz, estradiol, fentanyl, indinavir, HMG-CoA reductase inhibitors, (lovastatin, simvastatin), lidocaine, loratadine, methadone, midazolam, nimodipine, pimozide, prednisone, progesterone, propafenone, quetiapine, quinidine, ritonavir, sildenafil, tacrolimus, testosterone, tertiary amine TCAs, triazolam, vinblastine, warfarin, zolpidem, zaleplon, ziprasidone	Antifungals, calcium channel blockers, cimetidine, efavirenz, indinavir, fluvoxamine, fluoxetine, grapefruit juice, macrolide antibiotics, mibefradil, nefazodone, ritonavir, verapamil, voriconazole	Carbamazepine, glucocorticoids, modafinil, oxcarbazepine, phenobarbital, phenytoin, pioglitazone, rifampin, ritonavir, St John's Wort, troglitazone

CCB, calcium channel blocker; HMG-CoA, 3-hydroxy-3-methyl-glutaryl-CoA; mCPP, meta-chlorophenylpiperazine; NSAID, nonsteroidal anti-inflammatory drug; PPI, proton pump inhibitor; SSRI, selective serotonin reuptake inhibitor; TCA, tricyclic antidepressant.

REFERENCES

GENERAL NEUROLOGY

Aminoff MJ, Simon RR, Greenberg D. Lange *Clinical Neurology*, 5th ed. New York: McGraw-Hill; 2002: 271–274.

Cremens MC. Care of the geriatric patient. In: Stern TA, Fricchione GL, Cassem NH, et al, eds. *Massachusetts General Hospital Handbook of General Hospital Psychiatry*, 5th ed. Philadelphia: Mosby; 2004:447–456.

INDEX

N